REFLEXOLOGY

for Back Pain

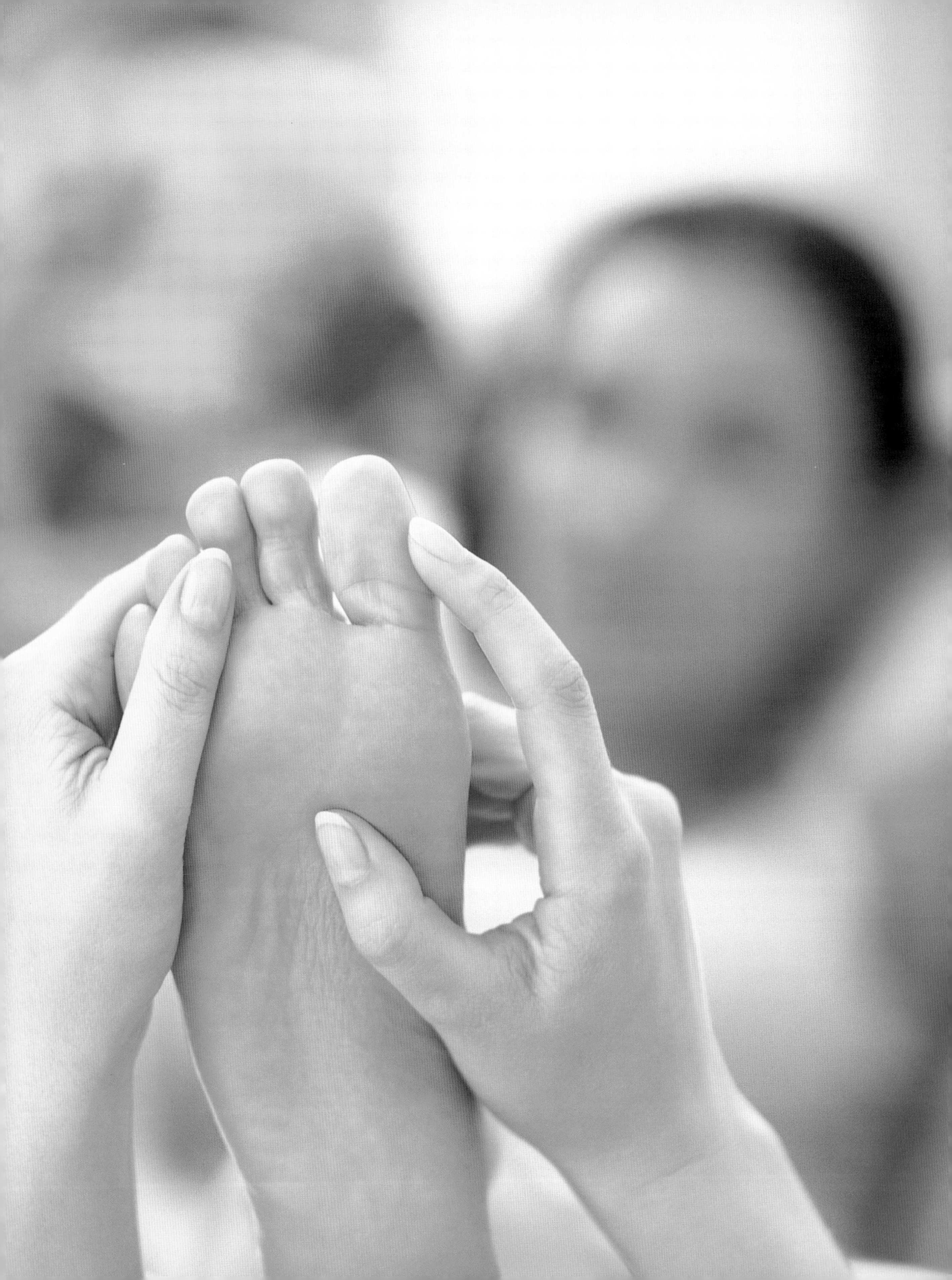

Ann Gillanders

REFLEXOLOGY for Back Pain

Healing your back in a safe and successful way

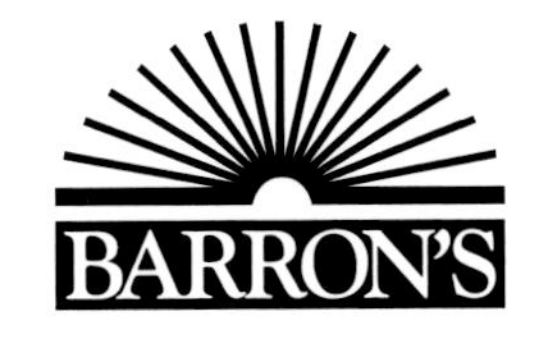

First edition for North America published by
Barron's Educational Series, Inc., 2005.

First published 2005 under the title *Reflexology for Back Pain*
by GAIA an imprint, part of Octopus Publishing Group Ltd
2-4 Heron Quays, Docklands, London E14 4JP

All inquiries should be addressed to:
Barron's Educational Series, Inc.
250 Wireless Boulevard
Hauppauge, NY 11788
www.barronseduc.com

International Standard Book No. 0-7641-3196-6
Library of Congress Catalog Card No: 2005920615

A GAIA ORIGINAL
Books from Gaia celebrate the vision of Gaia, the self-sustaining living Earth, and seek to help readers live in greater personal and planetary harmony.

Printed and bound in China

9 8 7 6 5 4 3 2 1

Caution

This book is not intended to replace medical care under the direct supervision of a qualified doctor. Before making any changes in your health regime, always consult your doctor.

Reflexology is a very safe therapy, but it's important to seek professional advice if you are in any doubt about a medical condition. Do not treat people who are suffering from any serious disease and always seek advice from a professional reflexologist before treating women during the first 14 weeks of pregnancy, particularly if they have a history of miscarriage. Any application of the ideas and information contained in this book is at the reader's sole discretion and risk.

DEDICATION

To my dear son Jonathan, whose birth and ensuing health problems led me into a career in a field of healing that I would never have dreamed possible

Author's Acknowledgments

I would like to thank Jinny Johnson for her untiring help and expertise in editing the text and Phil Gamble for his design skills and photographic excellence. The foot maps were developed in consultation with Jonathan Bispham DO (London) and I'd like to thank him for all his work.

ANN GILLANDERS

CONTENTS

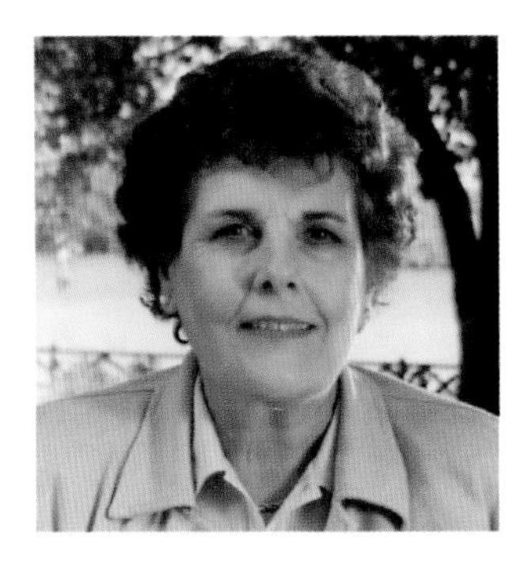

About this book

Easy to use and deeply relaxing, reflexology works to restore your body's power to heal itself. Simply by applying pressure to reflex points in the feet, you can remove blockages in energy pathways in the body and open the channels for natural healing.

I've been a practicing reflexologist for more than 30 years. I've treated thousands of patients with all sorts of conditions and I've trained many people in reflexology. Like many therapists, I find that one of the most common ailments I treat today is back pain, and I know that reflexology can bring relief to people suffering from all kinds of back problems.

With the help of this book you can learn how to use reflexology to ease back pain, as well as to promote and nourish a state of well-being in those you treat. Perhaps you might like to learn reflexology with a partner or friend so you can treat each other? Or perhaps you have a relative with a back condition you'd like to help? Whatever your situation, reflexology treatment is a pleasure both to give and receive.

Ann Gillanders.

Ann Gillanders

1 REFLEXOLOGY AND BACK HEALTH

Reflexology is a completely safe and highly effective method of healing. It works by applying pressure to specific reflex points on the feet. Each reflex point corresponds to a particular organ or part of the body (see pages 22–29). If there's a problem in your body, the reflex points in your feet will reveal a sensitivity. In this way, your feet can tell an accurate story about your health. When precise pressure is applied to the sensitive reflex, there's a stimulating effect through the nervous system. This reduces pain, improves nerve and blood supply, normalizes body functions, and relaxes the body, mind, and spirit.

Left and right sides

Everything on the right half of your body corresponds to reflex points on the right foot. Everything on the left half corresponds to the left foot. Imagine a line running down the center of your body from your head to your toes to help you keep this image in mind.

Reflexology is a "medicine of the soul." It reaches the very root of the physical or emotional problem and treats the sufferer holistically.

Healing is simple—it is humans who have complicated the process. The basic needs for healing are clean, fresh water, fresh air, a diet that is natural and as free as possible from additives, colorings, and preservatives, sufficient exercise, and space to roam in order to achieve stillness of mind.

The body wants to be well. It works hard to achieve a sense of balance and has remarkable powers for protecting itself against disease. Indeed, the workings of the human body are quite miraculous.

An ancient therapy

Reflexology is a noninvasive therapy that can be used to treat young and old. It dates back centuries. Ancient Egyptian paintings in the Tomb of Saquarra, known as The Physician's Tomb, show people treating each other by foot therapy, indicating that the therapeutic benefits were already well known. The inscription above them reads, "I shall act so that you praise me."

In the fourth century A.D. the Chinese are known to have used reflexology in conjunction with acupuncture. Dr. Wai Hong, a Chinese doctor of the time, found that applying pressure to the feet, once the needles were in place, helped to release energy and maximize healing. The therapy was introduced to the West in the 1930s by an American physiotherapist named Eunice Ingham, who learned about reflexology from ancient foot maps and refined its use for the modern world.

Who can benefit?

Reflexology can benefit people of all ages. The elderly, in particular, find the therapy very beneficial in relieving the aches and pains of rheumatism, arthritis, and so on. And older people who live by themselves and may be lonely, also draw great comfort from the healing power of touch. Reflexology can be used in conjunction with other therapies, including aromatherapy, massage, shiatsu, and homeopathy. By following the

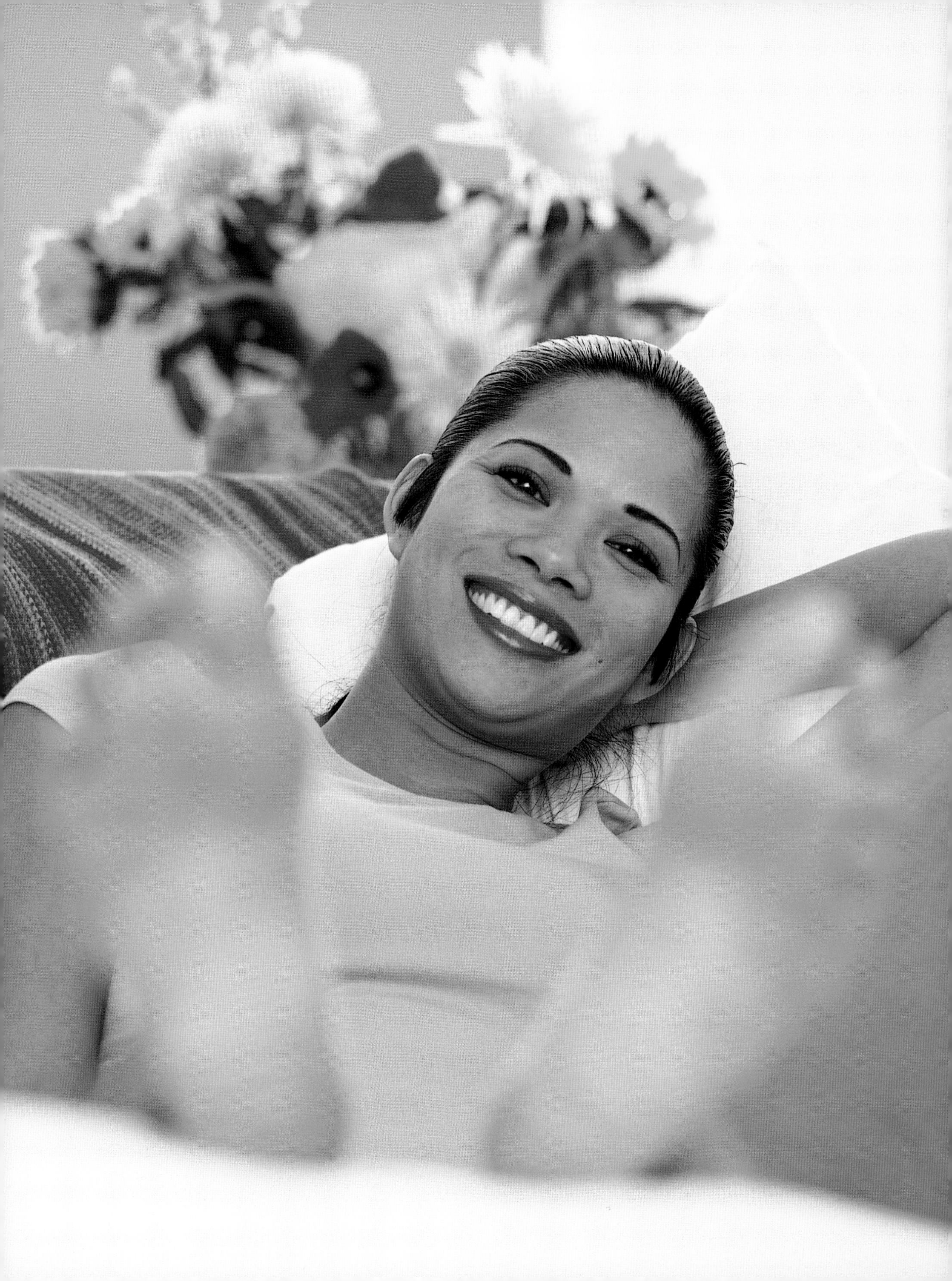

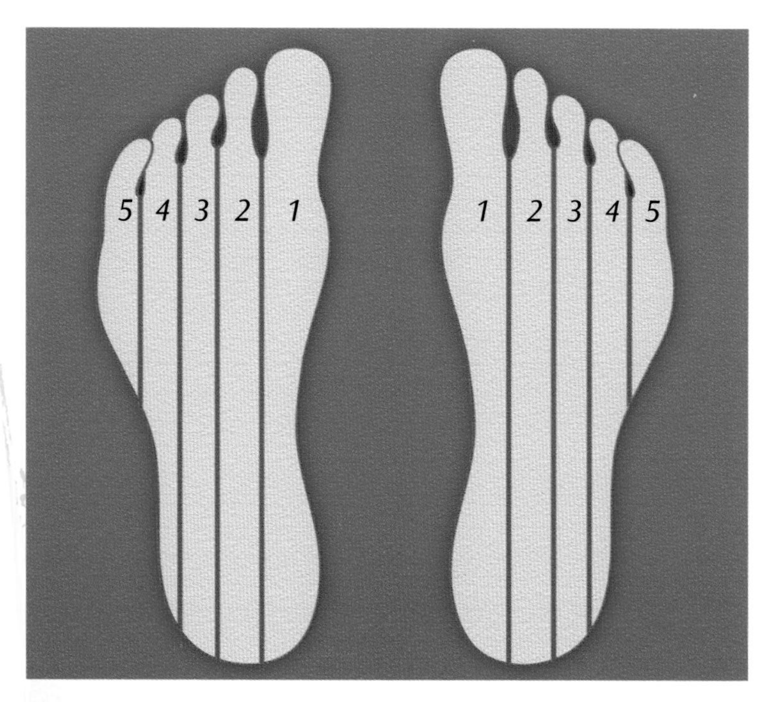

Energy zones

There are five energy zones on each foot. These correspond to the five zones on each side of the spine.
Zone 1: big toe
Zone 2: second toe
Zone 3: third toe
Zone 4: fourth toe
Zone 5: little toe

clear illustrations and explanations in this book, you'll be able to gain sufficient knowledge and confidence to help your friends and loved ones.

Energy zones

Visualizing the body's energy zones helps you understand how reflexology works. There are five pairs of energy pathways running through the body, beginning in the hands and feet and going up to the head. They are numbered one to five on each side of the spine. Reflexologists believe that any condition that interrupts the flow of energy in a zone disturbs the healthy functioning of the body parts lying along it. So if you apply pressure to the zones in the feet, the whole zone will be stimulated and the healing effects felt throughout the body.

Reflexology and back pain

Reflexologists and massage therapists treat more patients with back conditions than any other type of health problem. Reflexology is a wonderful therapy for people with back problems. Stiffness and disability, sciatica, lumbago, arthritis, whiplash injury, osteoporosis, and sports injuries are just a few of the conditions that respond well to treatment.

Disabling back pain strikes 80 percent of us at some time during our lives. It is second only to head pain in causing millions of work days lost and brings a steady stream of sufferers to doctors' offices and hospitals.

One reason why back pain is so common, and is on the increase, is that we have grown so much taller in such a short period of time. The average height for an adult is 1 to 1¼ inches (2.5 to 3 cm) more than it was 60 years ago.

Generally speaking, the taller you are, the more likely you are to suffer from back conditions, simply because the spine has more to support. In order for our spines to remain pain free, we need to be supported at both ends, like four-legged animals, once we reach 6 feet (1.8 m) or so in height.

A person with a shorter, fatter body has less trouble with back pain, as there is less "stretch" on the spine, plus the fact that when there's more body fat, there's a higher estrogen level. Estrogen helps to retain the mobility of our joints and a good level of calcium in bone.

The human skeleton

The living skeleton is a strong flexible structure. Made up of about 206 bones, it is the body's framework and has five main functions. These are to provide support, to protect organs inside the body, to work with muscles to allow movement to produce blood cells, and to store and release minerals such as calcium and phosphorus.

The skeleton can be divided into two main parts: the axial skeleton and the appendicular skeleton. The axial skeleton is the skull, spine, rib cage, and sternum and is the basic structure on to which the appendicular skeleton—the legs and arms—is joined via the pelvic and shoulder girdles. The pelvic girdle is particularly strong as it has to support the full weight of the body.

The skeleton is built up of different types of bones. There are the long bones from hip to knee and from shoulder to elbow, short bones in the fingers and toes, flat bones, such as the cranium, scapula, and pelvic region, and the irregularly shaped bones called vertebrae that make up the spine or backbone.

The spinal column itself works somewhat like a row of cotton reels strung on a rope. It is made up of five groups of vertebrae—seven cervical vertebrae, twelve thoracic vertebrae, five lumbar vertebrae, five sacral vertebrae and the four vertebrae of the coccyx. Each vertebra is covered with cartilage and the space between them is filled with a thick disc of fibrous cartilage with a center made of soft tissue. These discs between the vertebrae cushion and protect each joint and act as shock absorbers for the spine.

The spine's structure makes it amazingly flexible. We can bend forward, backward, to the right, to the left, rotate our head upon our neck, look down to the floor and up to the ceiling—and we make these movements hundreds of times each day.

The base of the spine is wedged at the pelvis by the sacroiliac joint, which is shaped somewhat like an arrow and is supported by strong muscles that go from the base to the top of the spine on either side. The spine depends on the strength of these muscles to give it added protection when subjected to accidents or injuries.

Disc damage

When these muscles become slack as we get older, or from lack of movement, the intervertebral joints and discs can suffer displacement. If there's excessive strain, the outer coating of one of these cushions may collapse so that part of the soft matter inside the disc extrudes. This can cause excruciating pain and is wrongly referred to as a "slipped disc."

Discs themselves do not cause pain because they have no nerves. It is the displacement of these discs, leading to pressure on the nerve roots that arise from either side of the spine, which causes the pain.

Intervertebral discs also wear and become thinner as we age. This is why old people become shorter—they lose the space between the joints of the spine. If a spine is in poor shape, a disc may be squeezed out of existence and eventually becomes a hardened rim of gristle.

A degenerated disc may prevent mobility of the two vertebrae it is intended to separate. This exerts pressure on a nerve root at a point where it leaves the spine to serve a distant part of the body. This squeezing pain may radiate down the leg in a condition known as sciatica.

To keep discs healthy you need at least a gram of calcium a day, as well as an adequate intake of vitamins D, C, and E. To help heal disc tissue, you'll need extra vitamin E.

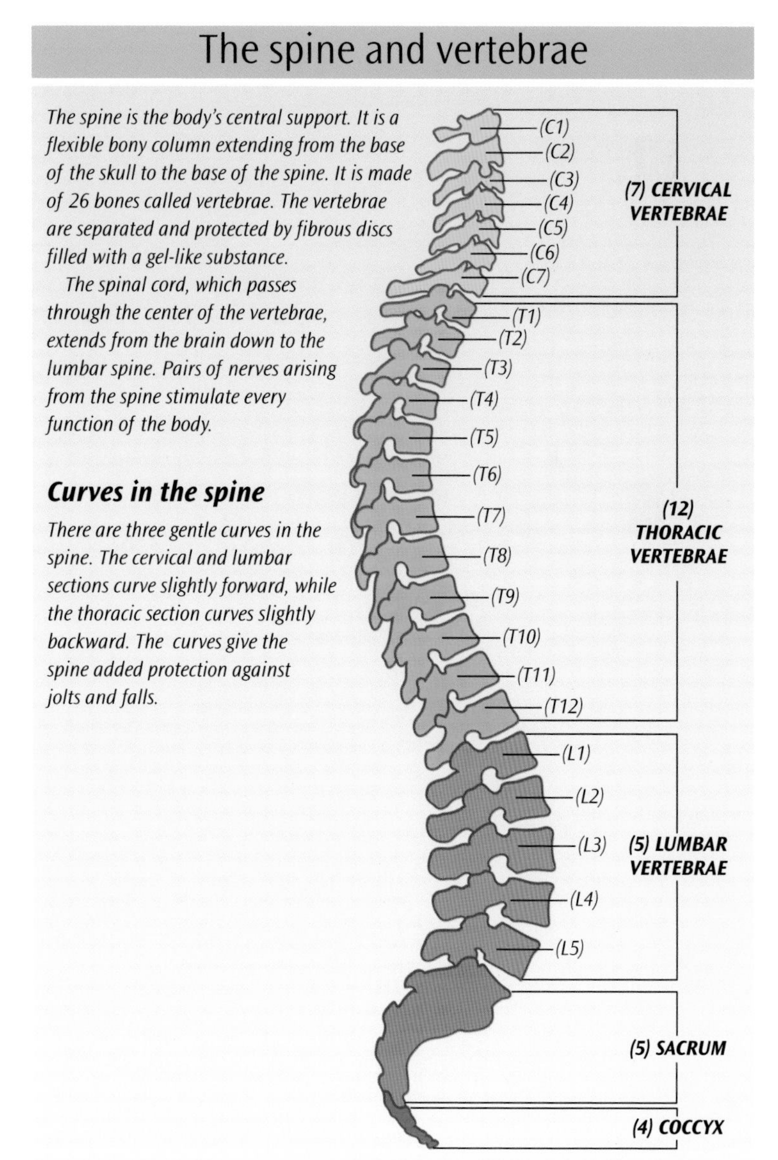

The spine and vertebrae

The spine is the body's central support. It is a flexible bony column extending from the base of the skull to the base of the spine. It is made of 26 bones called vertebrae. The vertebrae are separated and protected by fibrous discs filled with a gel-like substance.

The spinal cord, which passes through the center of the vertebrae, extends from the brain down to the lumbar spine. Pairs of nerves arising from the spine stimulate every function of the body.

Curves in the spine

There are three gentle curves in the spine. The cervical and lumbar sections curve slightly forward, while the thoracic section curves slightly backward. The curves give the spine added protection against jolts and falls.

Types and causes of back pain

Always warm up

To protect the back from injury, it's important always to do some gentle warm-up stretches before playing sports or doing vigorous exercise.

The two main causes of back pain are first, physical strains and stresses and their effects, and second, deterioration in the spine due to age or illnesses, such as arthritis. Back problems may also be caused by pregnancy and poor posture.

Physical strains and stresses

The function of muscles is to move the bones to which they are attached. They also work to hold one part of the body firm while another is moving. For example, the back muscles keep your body steady while you move your arms and legs. The places where two bones join are called joints and the bones at a joint are connected by ligaments. Ligaments can tear and cause pain if they are under excessive strain.

Trauma or overuse can easily damage tendons and the muscle, and this is a common reason for back pain. Damage to tendons is difficult to heal as there is far less blood supply surrounding a tendon than a muscle. If you "pull" a muscle it's very likely that some of the muscle fibers have been torn. This is common in the case of damage to the shoulder. Lifting something heavy in an awkward manner is usually the cause of the problem and the sufferer will find it difficult to lift his arm, or to rotate it in any direction, until the inflammation subsides and the damaged area heals.

Herbal remedies for rheumatoid arthritis

Many herbs have significant anti-inflammatory action and so are helpful in the treatment of rheumatoid arthritis.

- *Feverfew has long been used in the treatment of fever, arthritis, and migraine. It acts to reduce inflammation.*
- *Circumin, which is the yellow pigment of turmeric, also has significant anti-inflammatory action.*
- *Korean ginseng relieves some of the physical and mental fatigue associated with the illness.*
- *Devil's claw seems to relieve joint pain.*

Rheumatoid arthritis

Rheumatoid arthritis and osteoarthritis are similar in that they cause pain, disability, and often deformity of a limb or limbs, but they have different causes. Rheumatoid arthritis is an auto-immune disease, whereas osteoarthritis is generally caused by wear and tear in joints and is common in the older generation. Reflexology is beneficial for both conditions, since it breaks down pain levels and chronic inflammation and encourages the body to heal itself.

Rheumatoid arthritis is one of the most common of all crippling long-term diseases. It usually affects the smaller joints—particularly those of the hands, wrists, and feet—but can also affect the joints of the spine. The spine is usually affected last and most sufferers of this disease start by experiencing pain and disability in the neck, which radiates down the spine.

Your immune system normally helps to protect you against the invasion of infectious diseases, but in the case of rheumatoid arthritis, the body's immune system seems to work the opposite way. It attacks the joints, and in particular the lining of the joints, the synovial membranes, which enable joints and bones to move with ease.

The initial symptoms of rheumatoid arthritis may be the onset of a sudden fever, with symptoms similar to an attack of flu—temperature, aching joints, depression, and a general feeling of weakness. Those suffering with rheumatoid arthritis often complain that they feel exhausted and edgy. The condition can develop over a period of weeks or months and sometimes it can "burn itself out." Symptoms then disappear and may remain dormant for years.

Women are more prone to the disease, and this tendency may be due to some genetic factor carried by the female sex hormones. You're also more likely to suffer from this disease if your parents, grandparents, sisters, or brothers have the condition. Rheumatoid arthritis is not an old person's disease and usually affects people between the ages of 30 and 60.

In general, rheumatoid arthritis is not found in societies that eat more "primitive" unrefined foods, and it's more common in societies with a so-called Western diet. It tends to be more severe among Northern Europeans. Whether this is due to climate, genetic factors or to a localized infection nobody really knows as yet.

A diet rich in whole foods, vegetables, and fiber, with limited meat, sugar, refined carbohydrates, and saturated fat, does seem to be helpful for most sufferers. There also have been some links to particular food allergies, most commonly wheat, corn, milk and other dairy products, beef, and plants of the deadly nightshade family (tomato, potato, aubergine, peppers, and tobacco). Eating cold-water fish, such as mackerel, salmon, sardines, and herring, can reduce inflammation, or some people prefer to take a regular dose of cod liver oil. Vitamins C and E, zinc, and selenium can also help control the disease.

Orthodox approaches to controlling the pain and stiffness are aspirin in the first instance and then various pain-killing and anti-inflammatory drugs, which unfortunately have quite a drastic effect on the digestive system. There are herbal alternatives, which can ease discomfort.

Osteoarthritis

Osteoarthritis is a degenerative joint disease. It mainly affects the elderly and surveys have shown that 80 percent of people over the age of 50 have some degree of osteoarthritis.

Under the age of 45, osteoarthritis is more common in men. After the age of 45 it is ten times more common in women.

It is a less complicated disease than rheumatoid arthritis and easier to control, but once you have osteoarthritis, it's there for life. Weight-bearing joints are affected—the hips, knees and spine in particular—and as the disease progresses, the hands and feet suffer, too. Thankfully, due to great improvements in surgery, hip and knee replacements can be very successful and give sufferers years of mobility, if all attempts at other forms of orthodox or complementary treatments have failed.

The onset of osteoarthritis can be very gradual. Morning joint stiffness is often the first symptom. As the disease progresses, there is pain in moving, which is usually made worse by prolonged activity and relieved by rest.

Since we are all living much longer, our joints become subjected to more wear and tear. Just think how many times a day you move your arms and legs starting when you get out of bed, stand up, walk, bend, and so on.

The worst thing that most of us do to damage our joints is to become overweight. The heavier you are, the greater the strain on all your joints, and the joints in your hips, knees, and ankles, your weight-bearing joints will be the first to suffer. As we age our bones become thinner and less able to take any form of extra stress or strain.

The back in childhood

Bone density is laid down in childhood. A good diet and plenty of exercise through childhood builds a strong skeleton. Bad habits can cause back problems surprisingly early.

Scheurmans disease is a condition that affects the spine and is increasingly common in children today. It causes compression to the vertebrae when the bones are still soft, particularly during the early teens, and causes pain in both the cervical and lumbar spine.

The condition may be on the increase partly because of the poor diet of many children and teenagers, with high levels of fat and sugar, and low fiber content.

Poor seating at school desks and the carrying of heavy bags of books may be contributing factors.

Children who suffer asthma and have to take steroids lose calcium in their bones. Steroids affect bone density as do many pain-killing medications and anti-depressants.

Children suffering from diabetes or juvenile arthritis have a higher incidence of osteoporosis later in life.

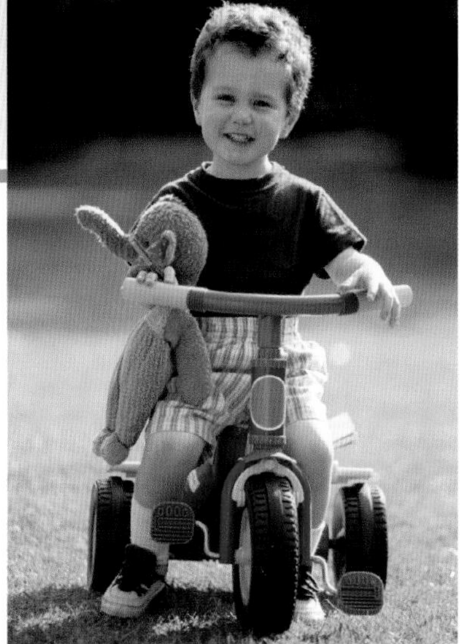

Pain is by far the most disabling symptom of osteoarthritis and can vary from a dull and persistent ache, to a sharp, gnawing pain. It is essential to keep moving—the longer you sit, the more stiffness and pain will result.

All the dietary, herbal, and mineral supplements mentioned for rheumatoid arthritis are worth trying for relief from osteoarthritic pain.

Sciatic pain

This affects the hip, buttock, leg, and back of the thigh, and pain can even radiate to the ankle. Indeed, sciatica is one of the most severe forms of back pain anyone can suffer. The cause is normally wear and tear of the discs in the lumbar spine. Because the sciatic nerve is the largest nerve in the body (as thick as your little finger), it is very difficult to calm it down once it becomes inflamed. Ice packs (see page 82) on the painful area are a great help and should be used several times a day.

Other causes of back pain

Lifting

If you bend over to lift a weight without bending your knees, you put a strain on the lumbar spine. It's not what you lift, but how you lift that matters. Always bend at your knees when lifting anything.

Lack of exercise

We need exercise to keep our bones in a healthy condition. Movement significantly improves our bones' ability to absorb calcium, but it must be regular. Try to walk briskly for at least 20 minutes every day and aim to do some stretching and toning exercise three times a week to prevent low back pain.

Anorexia

If you suffered from anorexia as a teenager you will have bone loss. Following a low-calorie diet for a long time has the same effect. The decrease in bone density will lead to back pain in later life.

Overexercising

Some young women dancers and athletes train to such an extent that their menstrual periods stop for a time. These women are particularly susceptible to fractures and back pain later in life because their normal oestrogen/progesterone balance has been seriously disrupted.

Gynecological problems

Back pain can be confused with gynecological problems. Women who've had several pregnancies may have a prolapse of the vaginal wall, which can cause back pain in later life. Check with your doctor about possible reasons for back pain.

Tips for easing back pain

- *If you suffer from back pain at night, waking after a few hours with discomfort in your lower back, try sleeping on your side and drawing up your knees as high as you can. This helps to stretch out the lumbar spine.*
- *Another tip is to have some chamomile tea with honey at bedtime, and avoid salty foods. Salt stimulates the adrenal glands, which in turn can irritate your muscles and create pain.*
- *An Epsom salts bath is an old-fashioned but effective remedy for back pain. Add two heaping tablespoons of Epsom salts to a hot bath to open up the pores and draw out inflammation. Always go straight to a warm bed afterward, otherwise you can easily get chilled.*
- *Lettuce leaves are an old remedy for soothing pain because of the traces of opium they contain. The effect is even more concentrated if you make a soup with plenty of lettuce thinnings, a sliced onion, and water or stock.*

Bad back?

Back pain is one of the most common reasons for time off work. Nearly everyone suffers back pain at some time in their lives.

Keeping your back healthy

Posture

The way we sit, stand and lie can have an effect on back health.

■ Try not to sit in the same position for a long time. Get up and move around at regular intervals.

Sitting slouched over a computer for hours on end can cause pain in the shoulders, neck, and arms. If you work at a computer, try to make sure you sit directly facing it, with your eyes level with the monitor. If you are constantly looking up when typing, you will affect your neck muscles, and this in turn can cause not only neck pain, but headaches too.

■ If your job involves many hours of driving each day and low back pain is often troublesome, get yourself a small pillow that fits neatly into the small of your back and gives you support. There are some very good orthopedic lumbar support pillows on the market, specifically designed for this purpose.

■ Try to "walk tall." Imagine you are trying to balance something on top of your head.

■ Make sure your bed is comfortable and supportive. Some people find that a board under the mattress helps to keep the spine straight and eases back problems.

■ Sleeping in a hammock is surprisingly comfortable. A hammock holds the spine in a semiflexed position, offering maximum relief, and the gentle swaying from side to side relaxes the pelvis.

Wear the right shoes

The type of shoes you wear affects the health of your spine, particularly during teenage/young adult years.

Very high-heeled shoes with narrow toes throw the weight of the body onto the toes, instead of the weight-bearing "platforms"—our heels. This encourages you to stoop over and increases the pressure on the lumbar spine. High-heeled shoes are fine for special occasions, but it's best to wear flat shoes, with plenty of space for your toes to move, whenever possible. Sneakers are very good for the comfort of your feet and help toward good posture.

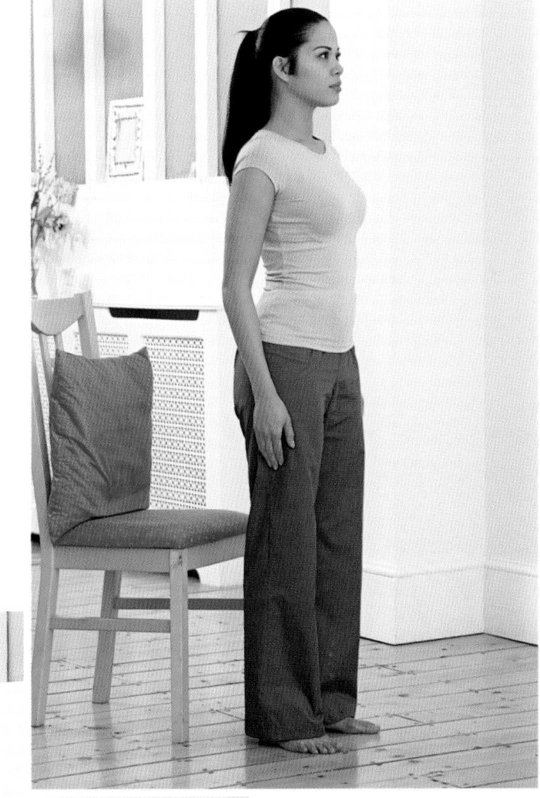

Stand tall

Try to stand tall. As you stand and walk, imagine you are balancing a book on top of your head.

Sitting

Choose a comfortable chair that supports your spine. Sit well back on the seat with your back straight and your head balanced over your hips. Don't slump.

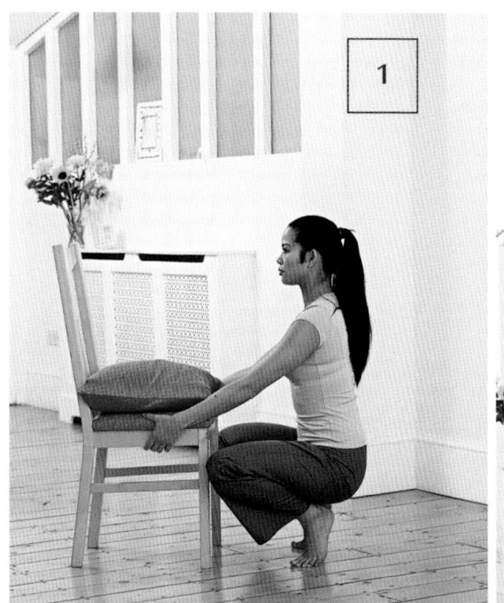

1. Squat down

Don't bend from your waist. Bending at your knees, squat down close to the object and hold it at the base.

2. Stand up

Keeping your back straight, stand up carefully, using the strength of your leg muscles not your back, and holding the object close to your body.

3. Stand straight

When you're standing up, keep the object close to you. Keep your back straight and your body well balanced, so as not to strain your back.

Take care of your back

Here are a few golden rules for back health:

- Cut down on coffee and alcohol and stop smoking. All reduce your body's ability to absorb calcium. Smoking also affects the blood flow to the spine.
- Aim for a diet that's high in vegetables and fruit and low in fat and animal products. Vegetarians generally suffer less bone loss than meat eaters.
- Aim to lose some weight if you need to. Being overweight puts a constant strain on your back. Try carrying a big bag of potatoes around with you for a while and see how stressful that is for your spine.
- Walk regularly and do some moderate physical exercise at least three times a week.
- Get a rocking chair. The gentle backward and forward movement can be very soothing and relieves a taut, exhausted back. Experiments show that the transmission of pain is blocked as long as rocking continues.
- When you lift something, place your feet as close to the object as possible, bend your knees and keep your shoulders back. Lift with your legs and not with your back. This safe way of lifting takes the pressure off your lower spine.
- When bending down to the bottom drawer of your filing cabinet, remember never stoop—squat or kneel instead.
- Check your car seat. Most car seats are badly designed and are responsible for millions of cases of backache. Make sure your car seat is properly positioned. If it's too far from the steering wheel you will strain your back and shoulder muscles. Adjust your car seat so that you can reach the controls comfortably without stretching. When making very long trips, stop at regular intervals, get out of the car, and walk around for a few minutes.

  If possible, fit a head restraint to your car seat to protect you from whiplash injury in the event of an accident.
- Keep your back warm. During the winter months try not to have a gap between your pants or skirt and your sweater. Letting this area get cold can cause the muscles in your spine to go into spasm and be painful.

Eating for a healthy back

Foods that are as natural as possible are the key to good health, including a healthy back. Eat plenty of fresh fruit and vegetables, as well as legumes, whole grain bread, and rice. Avoid deep-fried and processed foods, most of which contain a lot of salt, saturated fats, and artificial preservatives. Avoid eating too much sugar since this weakens the immune system and depletes bone density.

Build bone density

Teenagers aren't known for thinking ahead, but the teen years are the time for building healthy bones. Exercising and having a healthy diet with lots of calcium, as a teenager reduces your risk of back problems, osteoporosis, and fractures in later life.

Between the ages of 20 and 35 people tend to take fitness and good health for granted, but this is the time to build up a fit, healthy body so you're less likely to have back problems later.

At this age you are still building bone until peak bone mass is reached at around the age of 35. The higher your bone mass, the less likely you are to suffer from osteoporosis.

As we get older, bone density starts to decline and if you haven't built bone mass earlier, that's when problems start. Our metabolism tends to slow down, and if we are not very active, weight gain becomes a problem and can make back pain worse. You really need to reduce your intake by about 300 calories a day to maintain a steady weight if you're not able to be actively engaged in regular brisk walking, or some other form of sporting activity.

Calcium and magnesium

Calcium is the major constituent of bone and tooth minerals. The average human body contains about a kilogram of calcium and around a gram a day is needed to maintain that level. There's calcium in all dairy products, but these can be difficult to digest and cause sinus and respiratory troubles in many people. Also, too much protein in the form of milk, cheese and butter will actually cause a daily calcium loss. It's better to get your calcium in the form of sardines, almonds, soya beans, chickpeas, broccoli, spinach, and other dark green vegetables.

Magnesium helps muscle tone so it is another nutrient that's important for a healthy back. It's found in green vegetables and whole grains.

Avoid acid-making foods

All acid-making foods contribute to an acidic state in our blood and this will cause back pain. High on the list of acid-making foods are alcohol, red meats, high-sugar content foods, and white flour products.

Eat berries

Dark-colored berries, such as hawthorn berries, blackberries, blueberries, cherries, and raspberries, contain flavonoids (specifically, proanthocyanidins and anthocyanidins), which have a remarkable ability to stabilize and strengthen collagen in the body. Since collagen is the major protein structure in bone, it's important to keep up healthy levels.

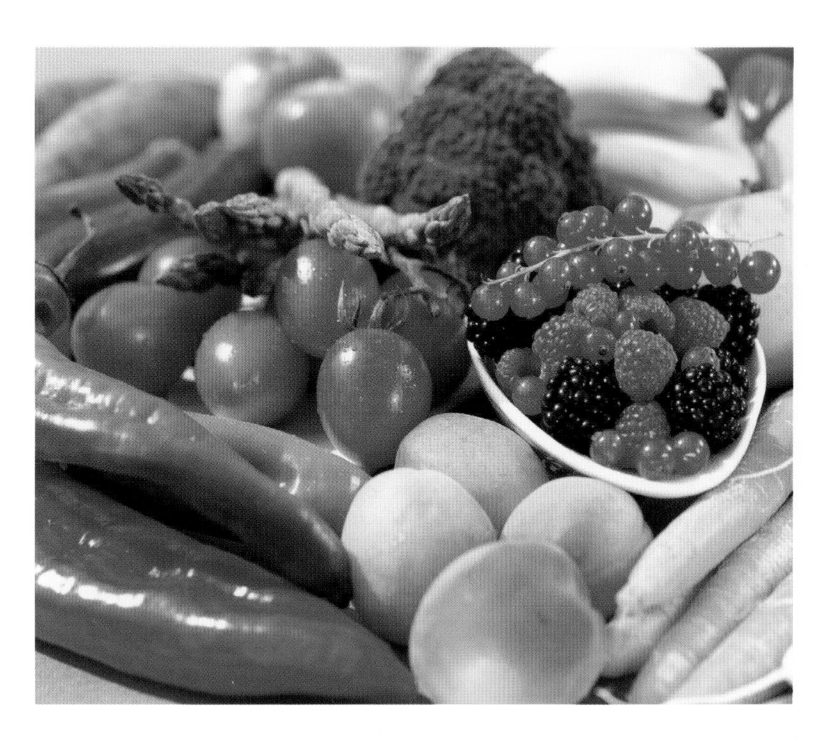

VITAMIN AND MINERAL SUPPLEMENTS

To aid the health of your bones, take the following supplements.

Recommended daily intake:
Calcium: 1g
Magnesium: 500mg
Pyridoxine: 100mg
Folic acid: 1mg
Vitamin B12: 1mg

Starting reflexology

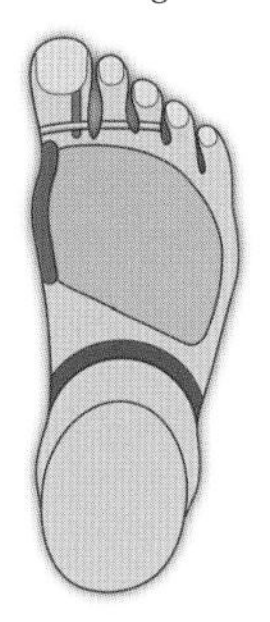

*The **plantar** side of the foot is the sole—the part you plant on the ground.*

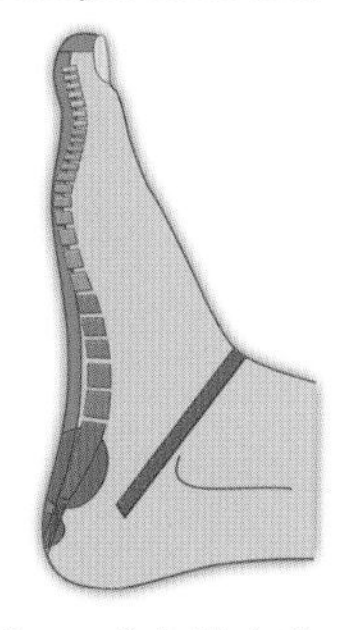

*The **dorsal** side is the top of the foot—the part you see when you look down.*

*The **medial** side is the inside edge of the foot, in line with your big toe.*

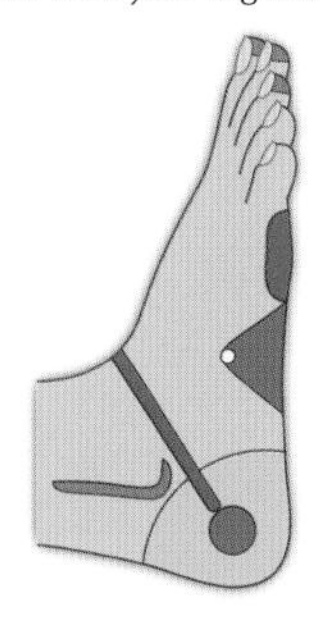

*The **lateral** side is the outside edge of the foot, in line with your little toe.*

Giving and receiving treatment

You and your partner or a friend could alternate giving and receiving treatment. Sharing time and physical contact with someone close to you like this is a healing experience in itself, and immensely rewarding.

Ideally, the room where the treatment takes place should be warm and pleasant. The receiver should sit in a comfortable chair with his or her legs up and feet supported on a cushion on the giver's lap. Otherwise, you don't need any special equipment—just your hands. Soften the feet with a little moisturizer first if you like, but don't use too much or the feet will be slippery. Never use oils—they make it hard to contact the reflexes of the feet properly. Before giving a treatment, make sure your hands are clean and your nails are short and well trimmed. This is important—long or jagged nails would be very uncomfortable for the receiver.

The basic techniques

Four basic techniques are used in reflexology. These are creeping, hooking out, rotating, and spinal friction. Experiment with these and practice until you feel confident that you've mastered each one.

The amount of pressure you use when giving a treatment depends on the individual and some people like more pressure than others. You need to exert enough for the receiver to feel reaction in the reflex points, but not so much that it causes pain. Generally, a healthy person can take a firmer pressure than someone who is elderly or ill.

Always work the reflexes on the right foot first and then move on to the left. Unless otherwise directed, treat each reflex area twice, working from the medial side to the lateral first and then working back from lateral to medial. For back pain, it's helpful to have a full treatment at least a couple of times a week.

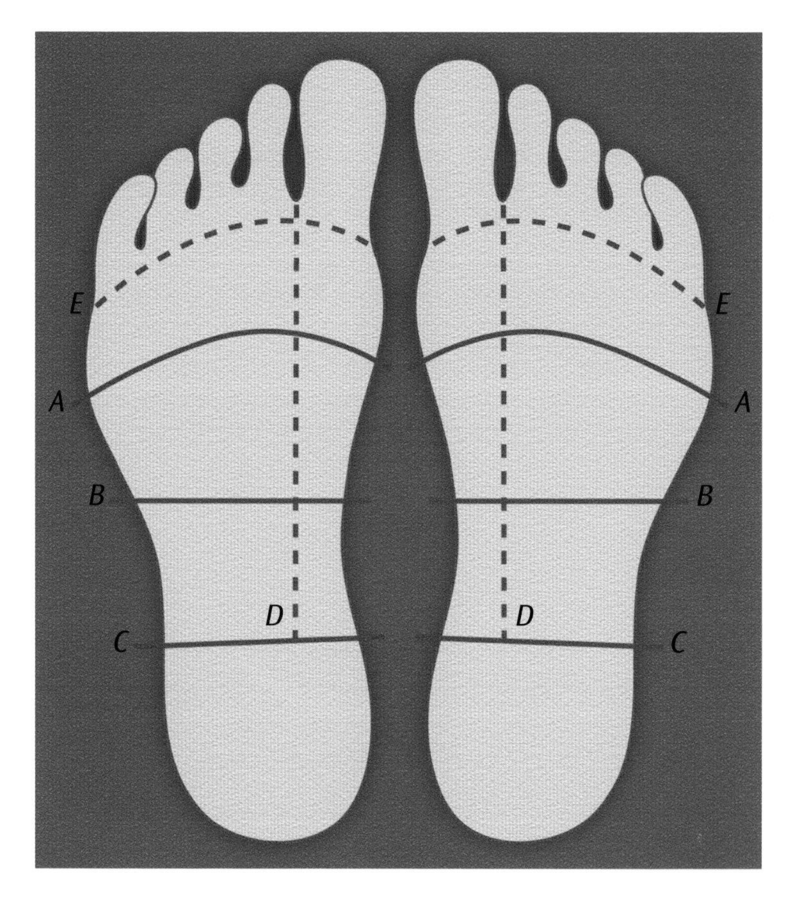

Foot guidelines

These guidelines show which areas of the feet relate to which area of the body. All reflex points are found within these guidelines.
A: Diaphragm line
B: Waist line
C: Pelvic line
D: Ligament line
E: Shoulder line

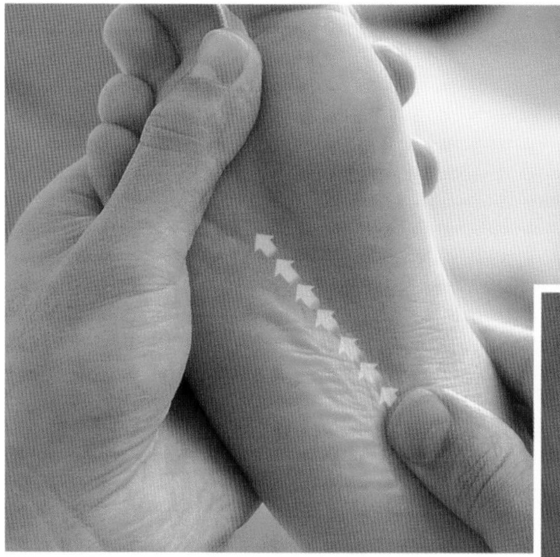

Creeping 1

In this technique, you move your thumb or finger forward in a creeping movement, similar to the way a caterpillar moves. Keep your thumb flexed and work with the flat pad. Press down slightly on the outer edge so that your nail does not dig in.

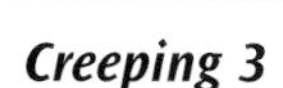

Creeping 2

Move your thumb across the foot with a tiny action that is slow and methodical.

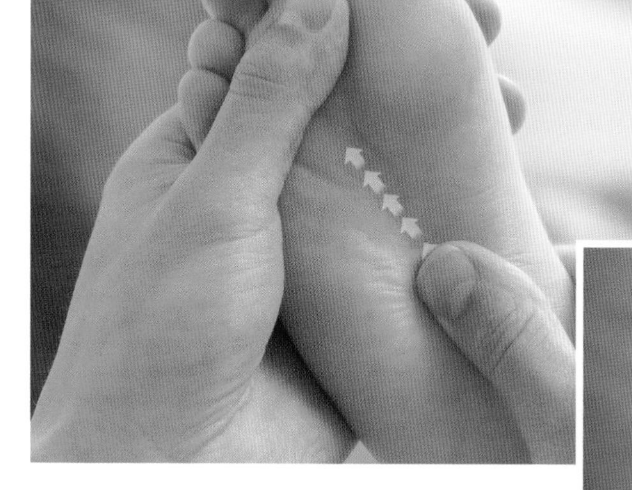

Creeping 3

As you move your thumb, imagine that you're working across a pincushion full of pins. Each time you lift your thumb, creep it forward and press down as if you were pushing one of the pins into the pincushion. Keep your movements as small as possible.

Creeping 4

The creeping movement is always forward, never backward.

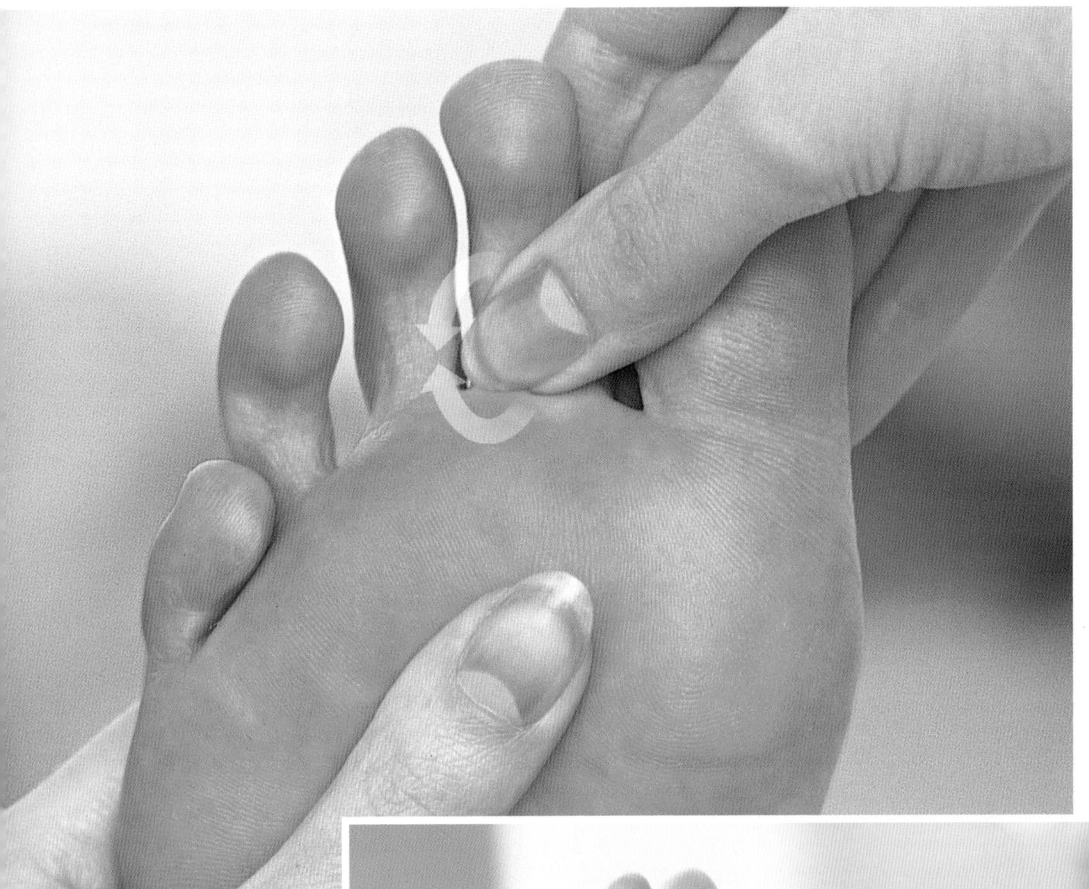

Rotating

For this technique, place the flat part of your thumb on the reflex point you want to work. With a small but firm movement, rotate your thumb inward, toward the spine. Keep up the pressure for several seconds for the greatest benefit.

Spinal friction

This special technique helps to stimulate and warm the spinal column. Place the palm of your hand on the inside edge of the foot and rub it up and down vigorously.

Overgrip

When working on the right foot, place the left hand on the ankle with your thumb on the outside. Using your right hand, turn the foot inward. Switch hands for the left foot.

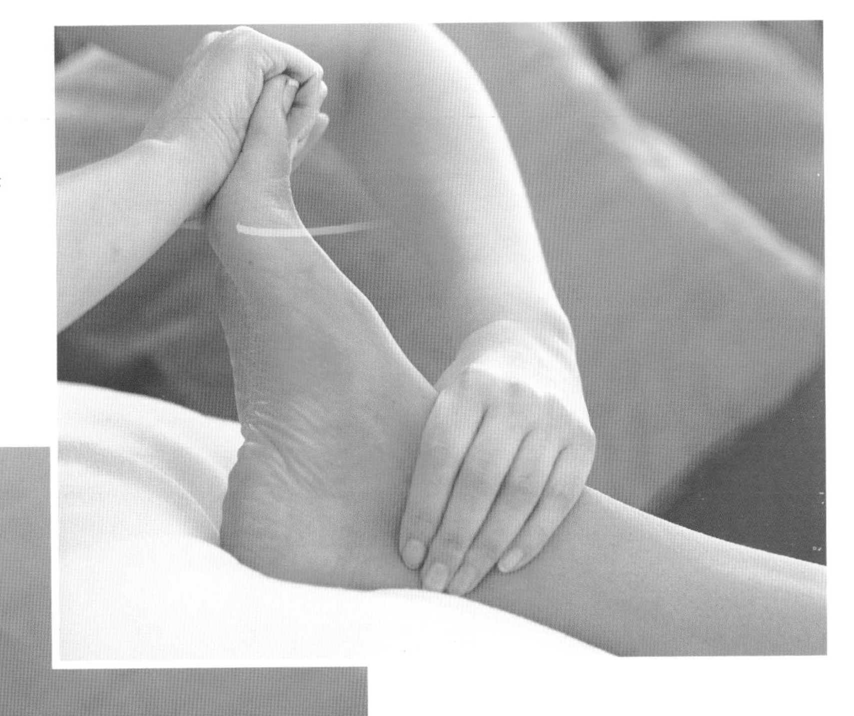

Undergrip

When working on the right foot, support the heel of the foot in the palm of the left hand. Using the right hand, turn the foot inward. Switch hands for the left foot.

Hooking out

This technique is used for extra stimulation of the ileocecal valve (the join of the large and small intestines), which is located on the lateral edge of the foot, near the pelvic line (see page 18). Using your left thumb, press down firmly on this point. With the flat of your thumb, make an outward-hooking movement in the shape of the letter "j". Hooking out is also used for working the eye and ear reflexes.

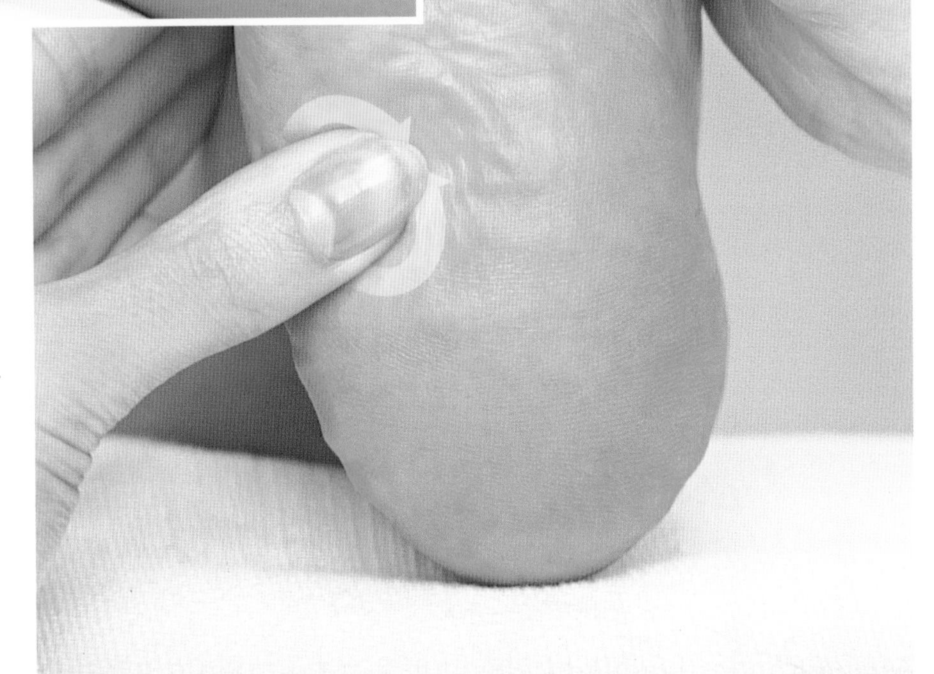

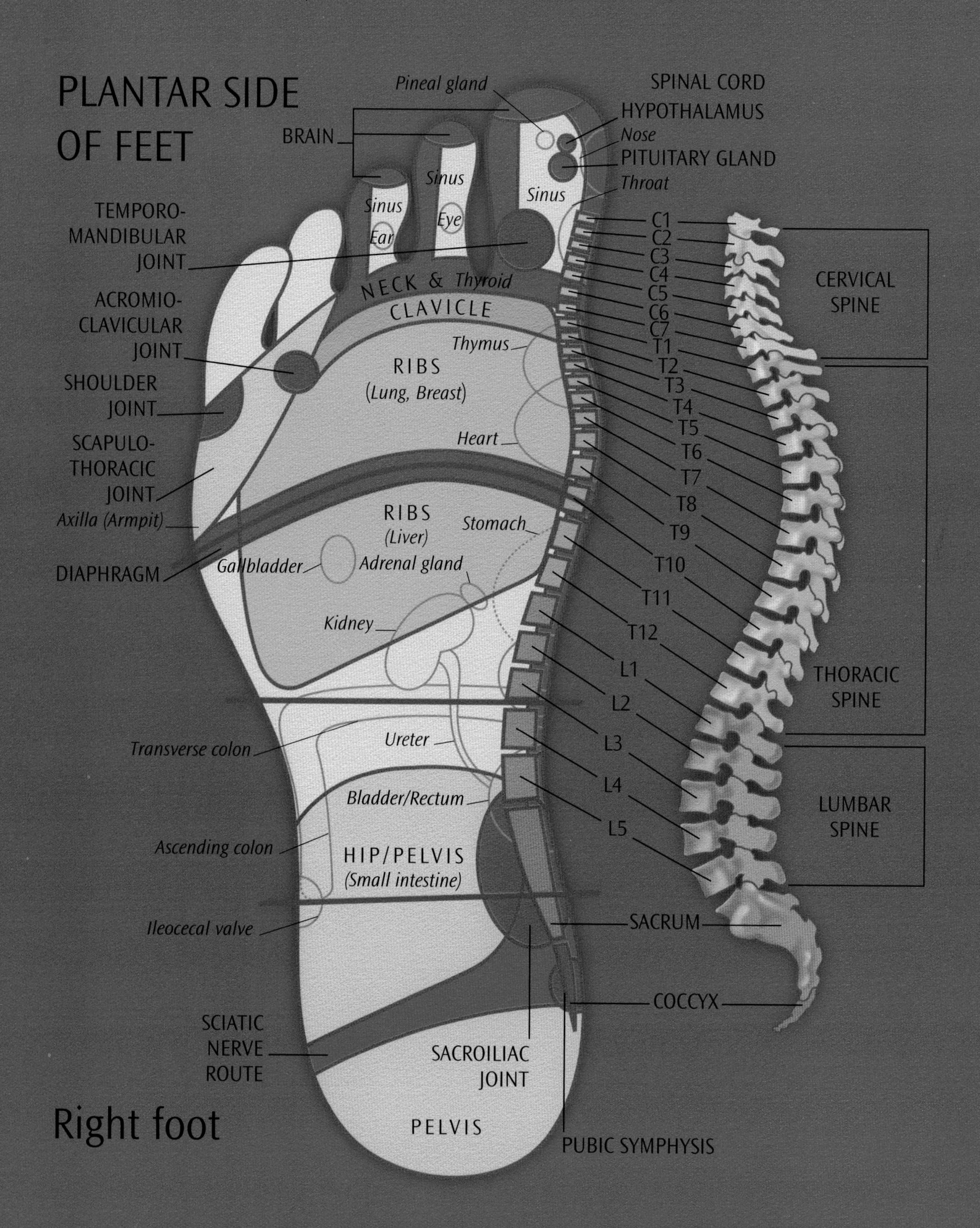

PLANTAR SIDE OF FEET
BRAIN
Pineal gland
SPINAL CORD
HYPOTHALAMUS
Nose
PITUITARY GLAND
Throat
Sinus
Sinus
Sinus
Eye
Ear
TEMPORO-MANDIBULAR JOINT
ACROMIO-CLAVICULAR JOINT
SHOULDER JOINT
SCAPULO-THORACIC JOINT
Axilla (Armpit)
DIAPHRAGM
NECK & Thyroid
CLAVICLE
Thymus
RIBS
(Lung, Breast)
Heart
RIBS
(Liver)
Stomach
Gallbladder
Adrenal gland
Kidney
Transverse colon
Ureter
Bladder/Rectum
Ascending colon
HIP/PELVIS
(Small intestine)
Ileocecal valve
SCIATIC NERVE ROUTE
SACROILIAC JOINT
PELVIS
C1
C2
C3
C4
C5
C6
C7
T1
T2
T3
T4
T5
T6
T7
T8
T9
T10
T11
T12
L1
L2
L3
L4
L5
SACRUM
COCCYX
PUBIC SYMPHYSIS
CERVICAL SPINE
THORACIC SPINE
LUMBAR SPINE

Right foot

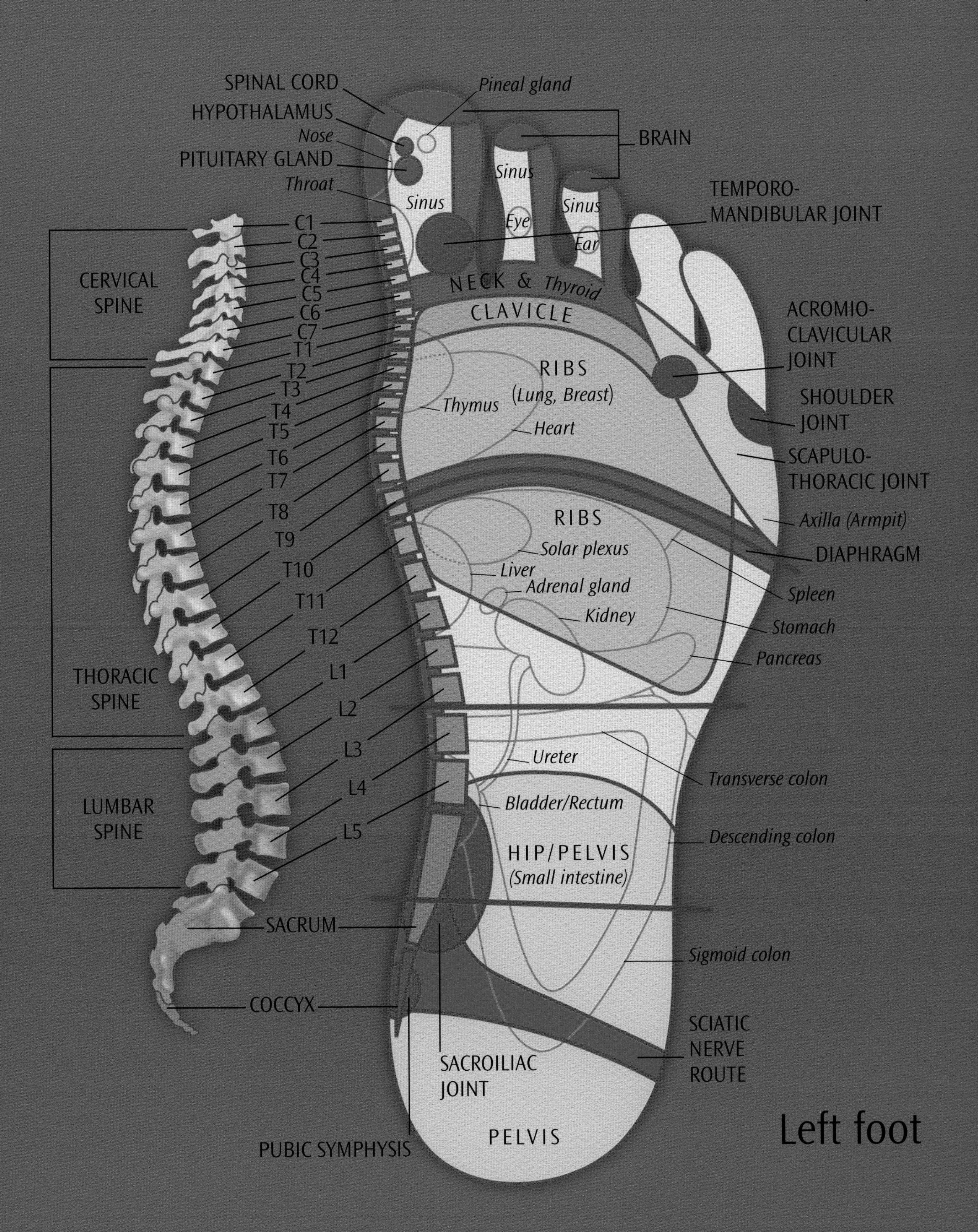
SPINAL CORD
HYPOTHALAMUS
Nose
PITUITARY GLAND
Throat
Pineal gland
BRAIN
Sinus
Sinus
Sinus
Eye
Ear
TEMPORO-MANDIBULAR JOINT
C1
C2
C3
C4
C5
C6
C7
T1
T2
T3
T4
T5
T6
T7
T8
T9
T10
T11
T12
L1
L2
L3
L4
L5
CERVICAL SPINE
THORACIC SPINE
LUMBAR SPINE
NECK & Thyroid
CLAVICLE
ACROMIO-CLAVICULAR JOINT
RIBS
(Lung, Breast)
Thymus
Heart
SHOULDER JOINT
SCAPULO-THORACIC JOINT
Axilla (Armpit)
RIBS
Solar plexus
DIAPHRAGM
Liver
Adrenal gland
Kidney
Spleen
Stomach
Pancreas
Ureter
Transverse colon
Bladder/Rectum
HIP/PELVIS
(Small intestine)
Descending colon
SACRUM
Sigmoid colon
COCCYX
SCIATIC NERVE ROUTE
SACROILIAC JOINT
PUBIC SYMPHYSIS
PELVIS

Left foot

DORSAL SIDE OF FEET

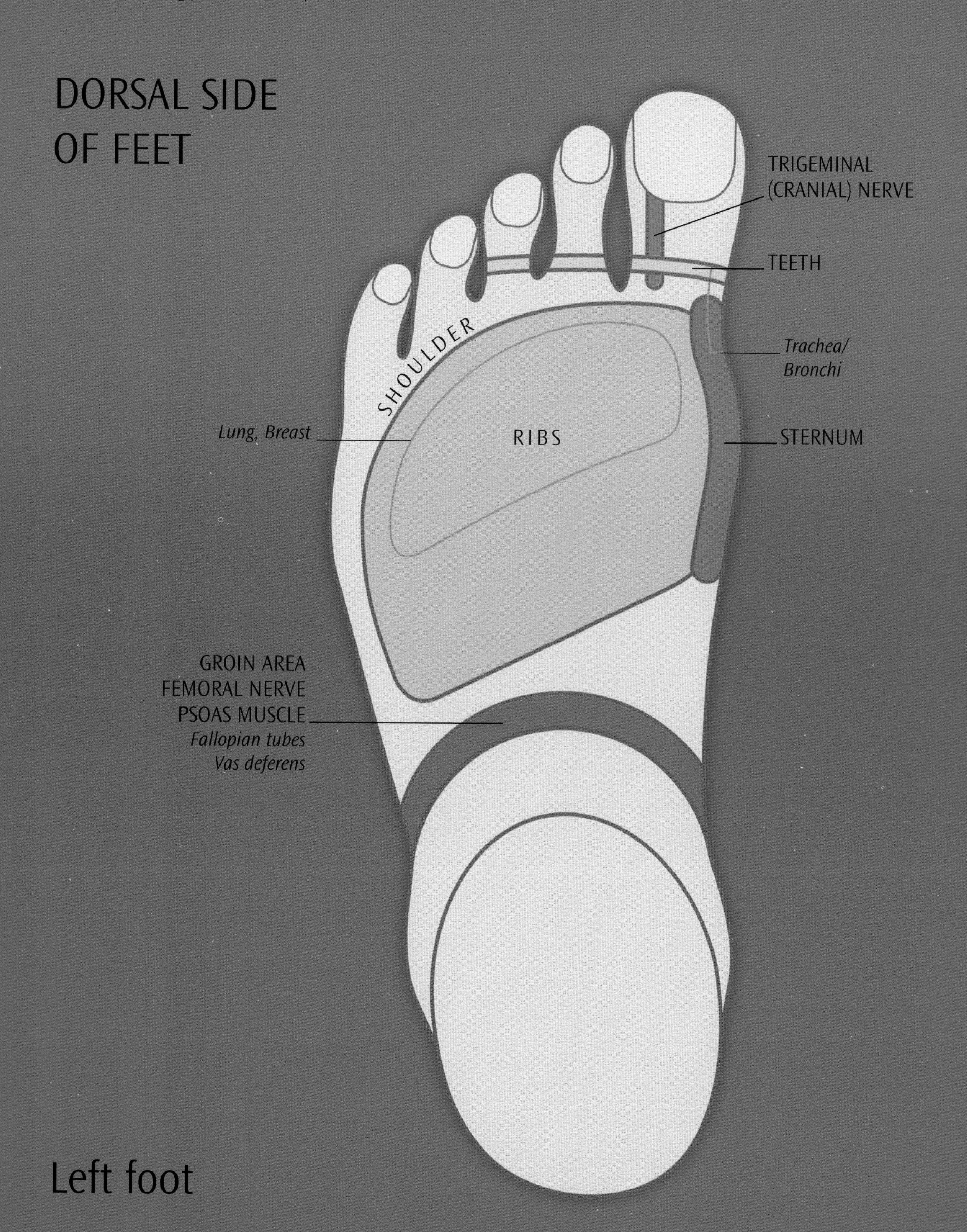

Left foot

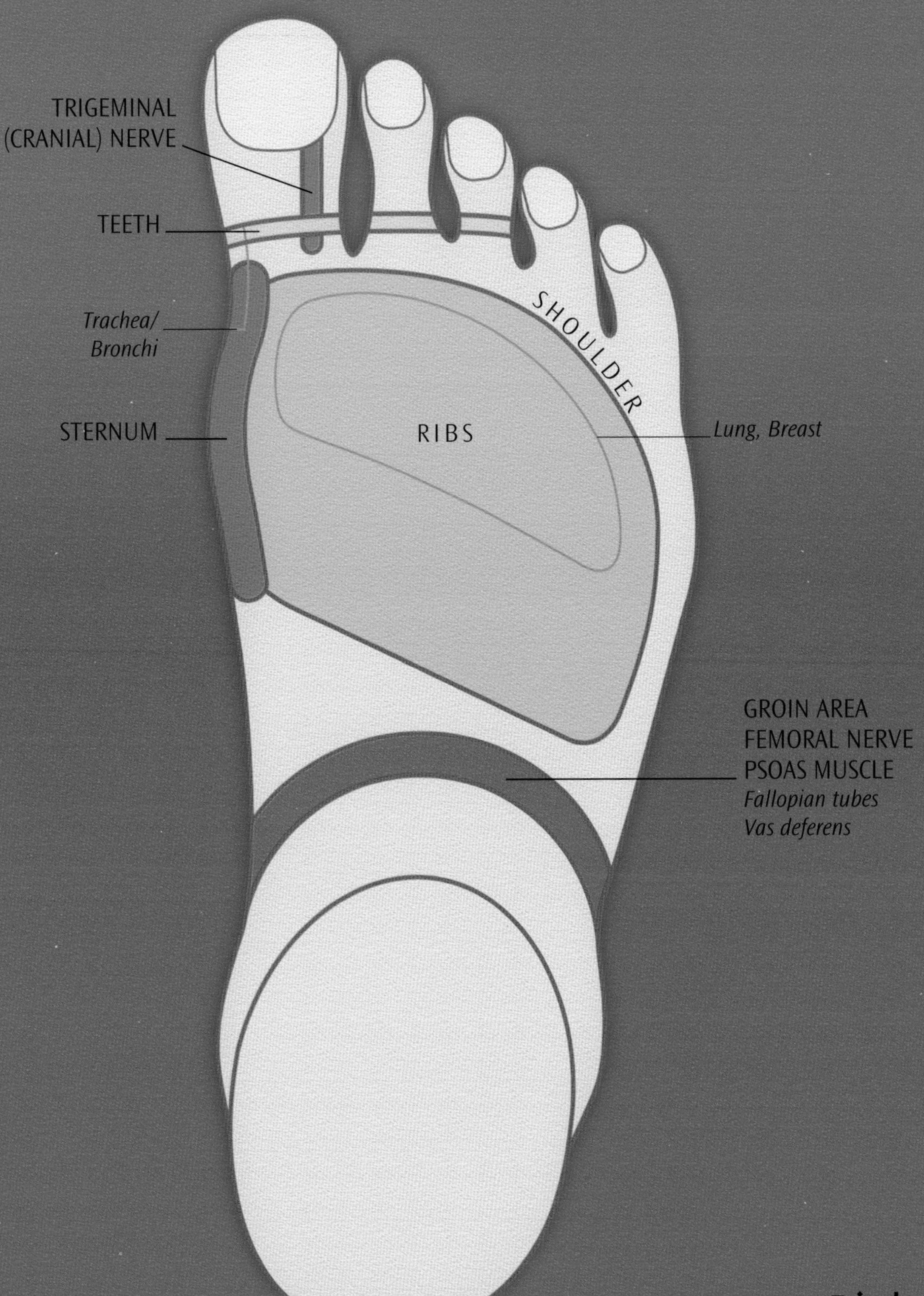
TRIGEMINAL
(CRANIAL) NERVE
TEETH
Trachea/
Bronchi
STERNUM
SHOULDER
RIBS
Lung, Breast
GROIN AREA
FEMORAL NERVE
PSOAS MUSCLE
Fallopian tubes
Vas deferens

Right foot

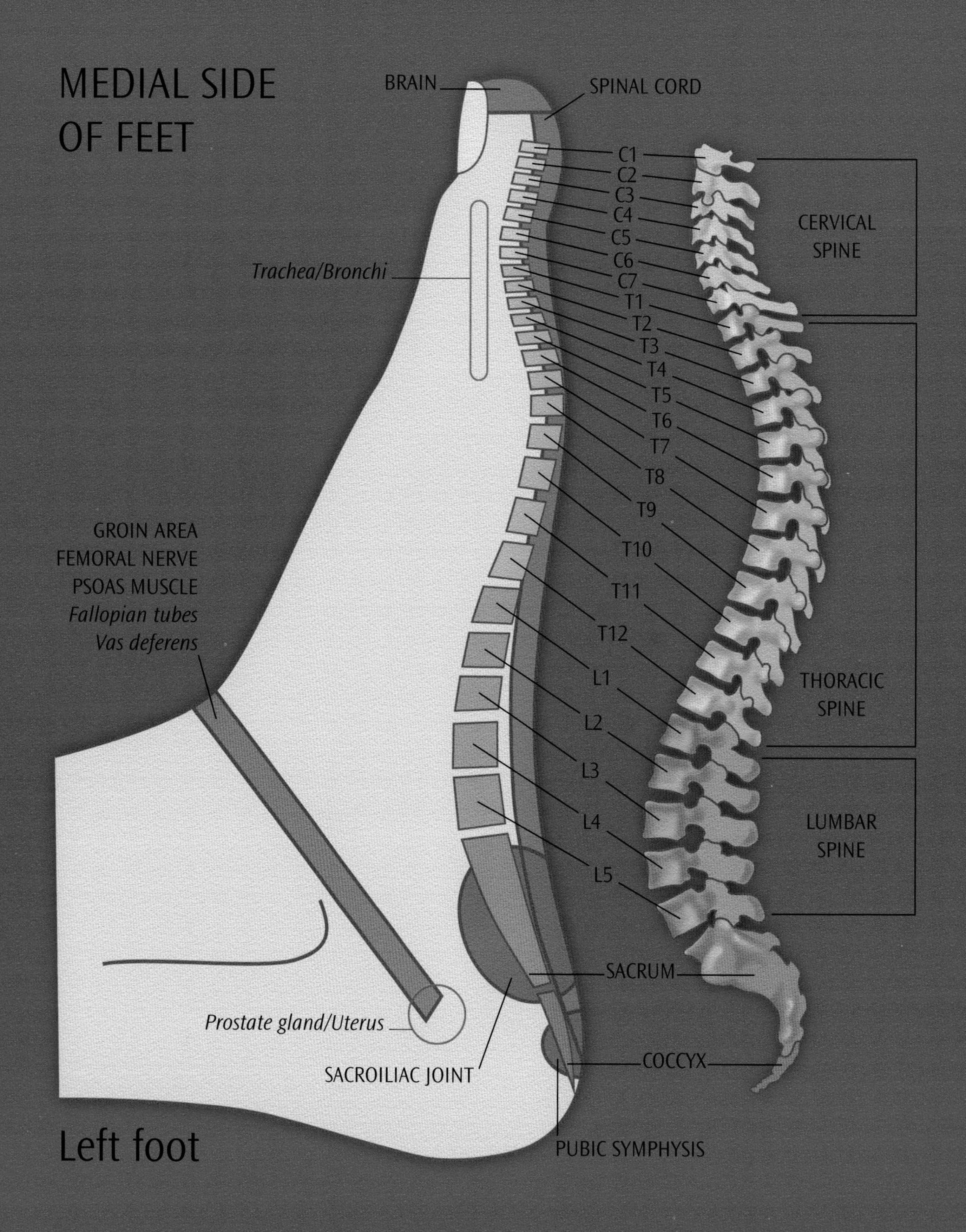
MEDIAL SIDE
OF FEET
BRAIN
SPINAL CORD
C1
C2
C3
C4
C5
C6
C7
T1
T2
T3
T4
T5
T6
T7
T8
T9
T10
T11
T12
L1
L2
L3
L4
L5
CERVICAL
SPINE
THORACIC
SPINE
LUMBAR
SPINE
Trachea/Bronchi
GROIN AREA
FEMORAL NERVE
PSOAS MUSCLE
Fallopian tubes
Vas deferens
SACRUM
Prostate gland/Uterus
COCCYX
SACROILIAC JOINT
PUBIC SYMPHYSIS
Left foot

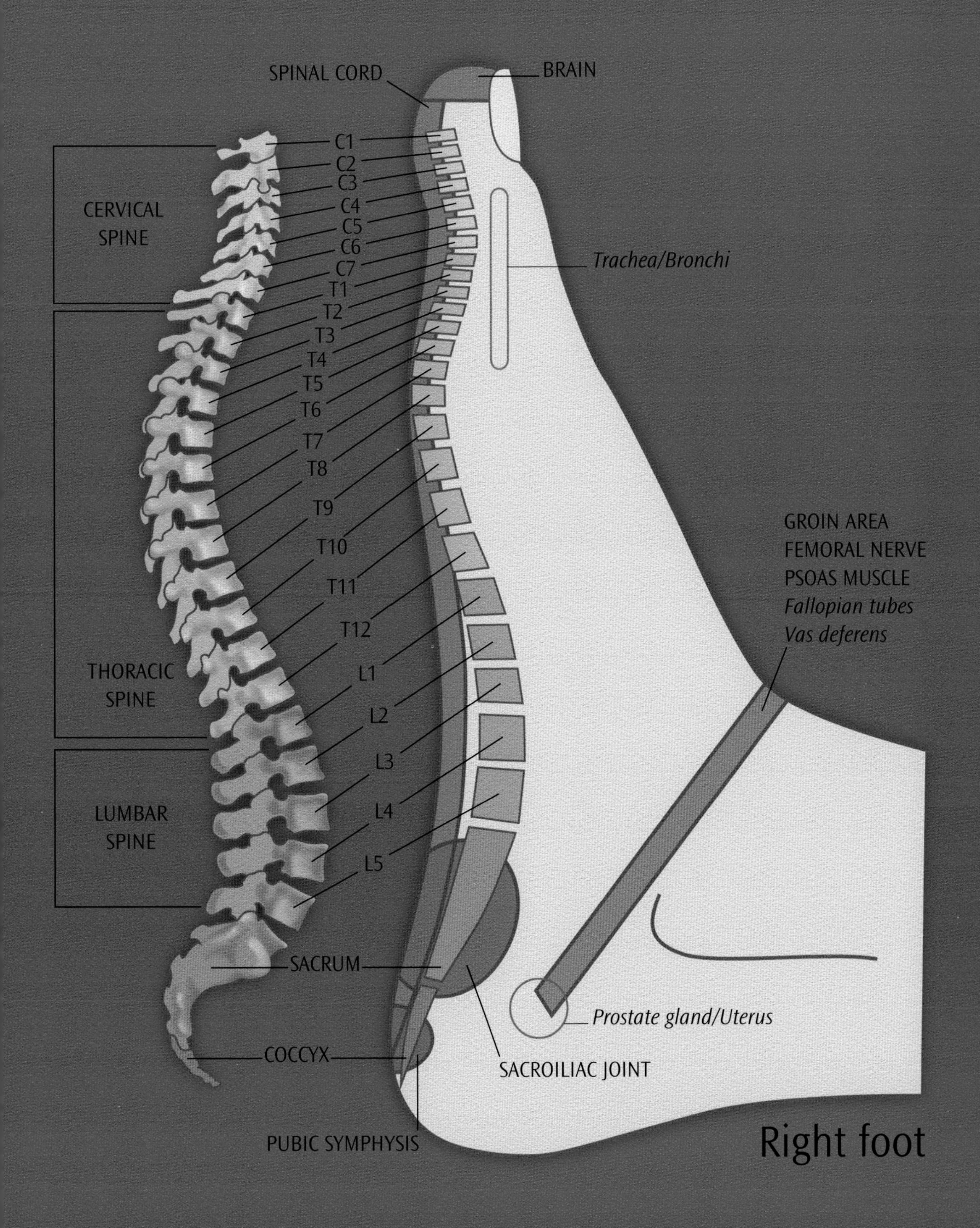
SPINAL CORD
BRAIN
C1
C2
C3
C4
C5
C6
C7
T1
T2
T3
T4
T5
T6
T7
T8
T9
T10
T11
T12
L1
L2
L3
L4
L5
CERVICAL SPINE
THORACIC SPINE
LUMBAR SPINE
Trachea/Bronchi
GROIN AREA
FEMORAL NERVE
PSOAS MUSCLE
Fallopian tubes
Vas deferens
SACRUM
COCCYX
Prostate gland/Uterus
SACROILIAC JOINT
PUBIC SYMPHYSIS

Right foot

LATERAL SIDE OF FEET

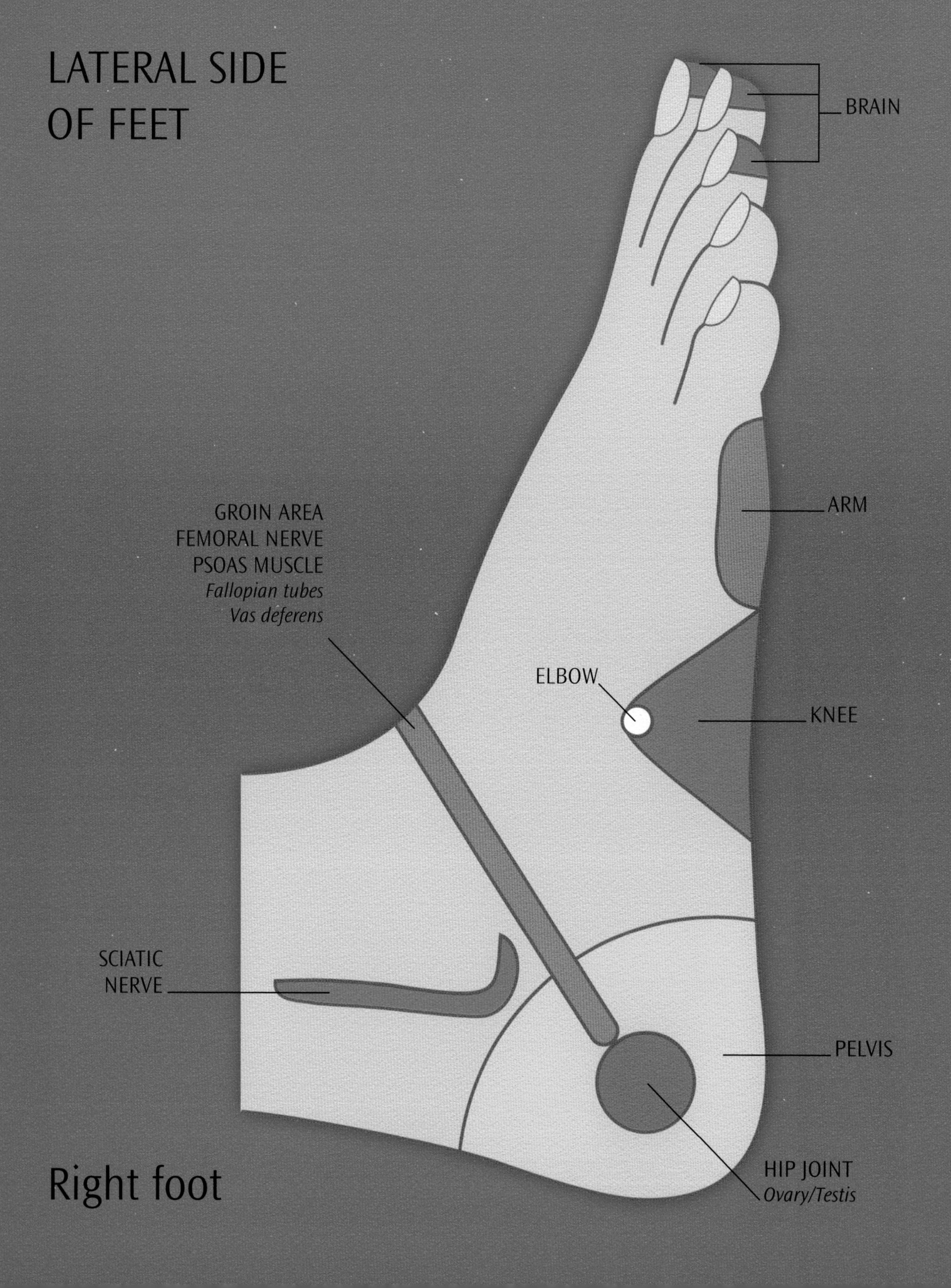

Right foot

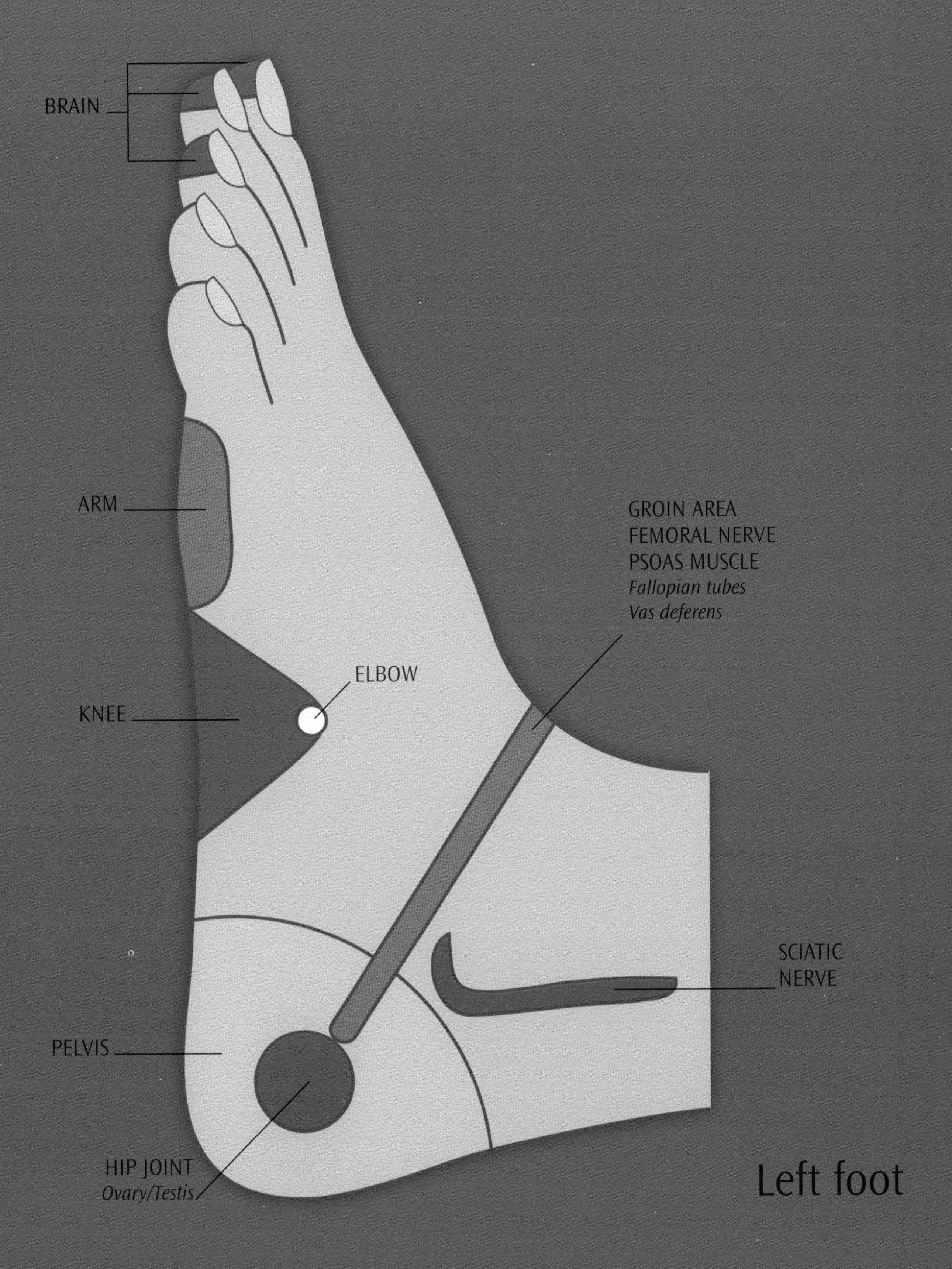
BRAIN
ARM
GROIN AREA
FEMORAL NERVE
PSOAS MUSCLE
Fallopian tubes
Vas deferens
ELBOW
KNEE
SCIATIC
NERVE
PELVIS
HIP JOINT
Ovary/Testis

Left foot

2 A COMPLETE FOOT SESSION

Reflexology is a holistic therapy, so when treating any kind of back pain, it's important to start by giving a full reflexology treatment for the whole body. This can be followed by work on the particular areas affected (see chapters 3 to 8).

A full treatment takes about 45 minutes. Both feet must be treated, regardless of which side of the body is suffering from pain and disability. Always start with the right foot and complete the whole sequence before treating the left. As a general rule, work on each reflex area twice. If any of the reflex points are particularly sensitive, work over them again.

Diaphragm relax

Starting with the right foot, place your right thumb on the start of the diaphragm line (see page 18). Pressing your thumb into the foot, work across to the lateral edge. At the same time, bend the foot onto your right thumb (1).

If the person receiving reflexology is tense and anxious, these feelings will be transmitted to the feet, making them harder to work on and more sensitive. For this reason, always start a treatment with foot relaxation exercises (see pages 30–39) to ease any tension in the receiver and help make the feet supple and flexible.

People new to reflexology may find these exercises a good way of getting used to handling the feet correctly. The relaxation exercises may also be used if you come across a particular sensitivity in the feet, or you can repeat two or three of them at any time during the reflexology session.

Ask the person receiving treatment to sit on a comfortable chair or even on a recliner such as a chaise lounge, with his or her feet on a large cushion on your lap. Some people like treatment to be carried out in silence; others prefer to see this as a time for chatting quietly and sharing their worries. Do whatever suits the receiver best.

A full foot treatment always gives the best results, but if you're short of time, or you're dealing with an emergency, you can just work the principal reflexes indicated for specific ailments. Choose what seems right to you or offer the treatments the receiver enjoys most.

After a full session you should notice that any tender reflex areas will have become less sensitive, making any further treatments more effective.

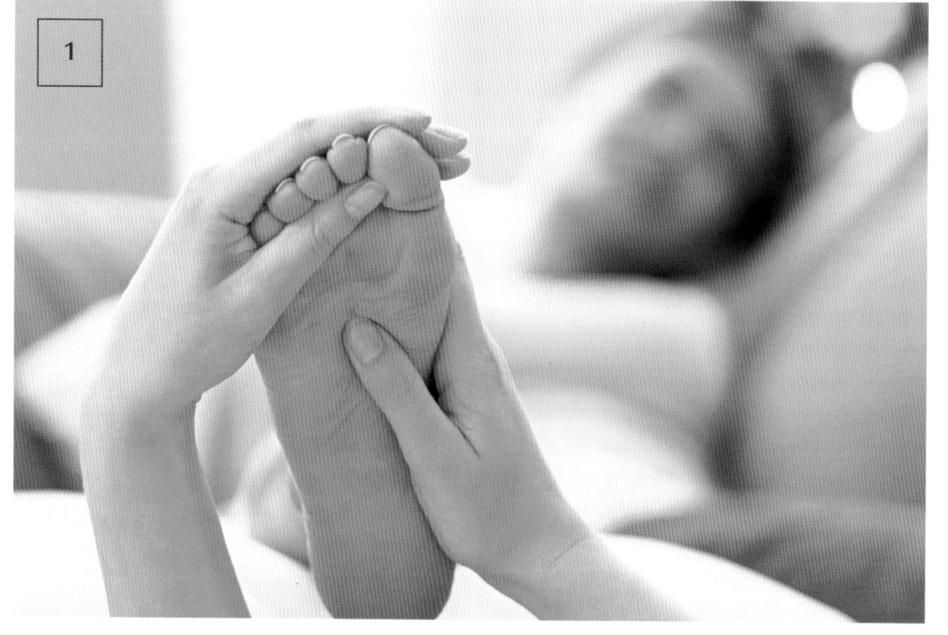

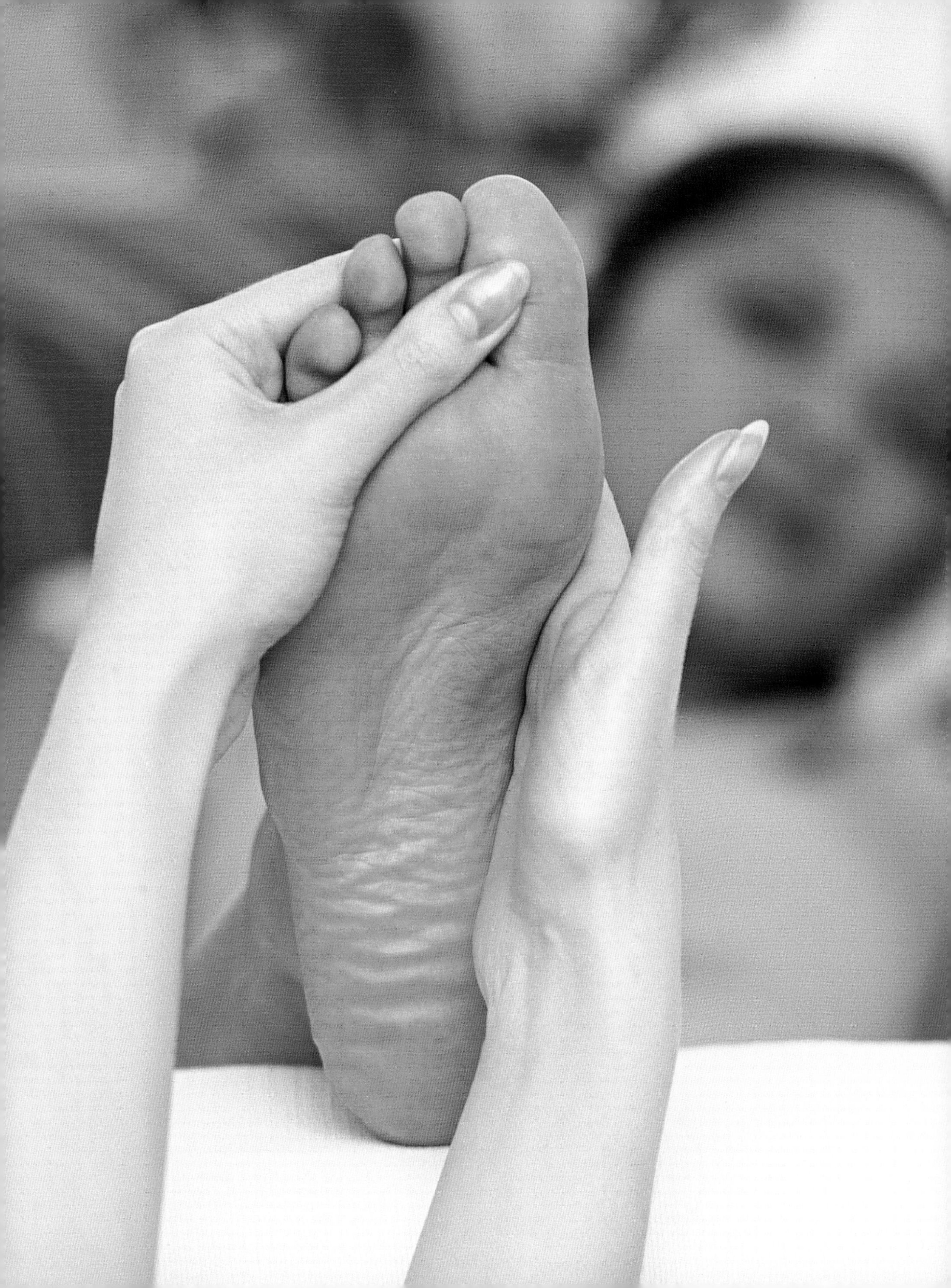

Side to side relax

Support the foot with both hands. Rock the foot from side to side between your palms, keeping your movements rapid but gentle (2A, 2B, 2C). Repeat with the other foot.

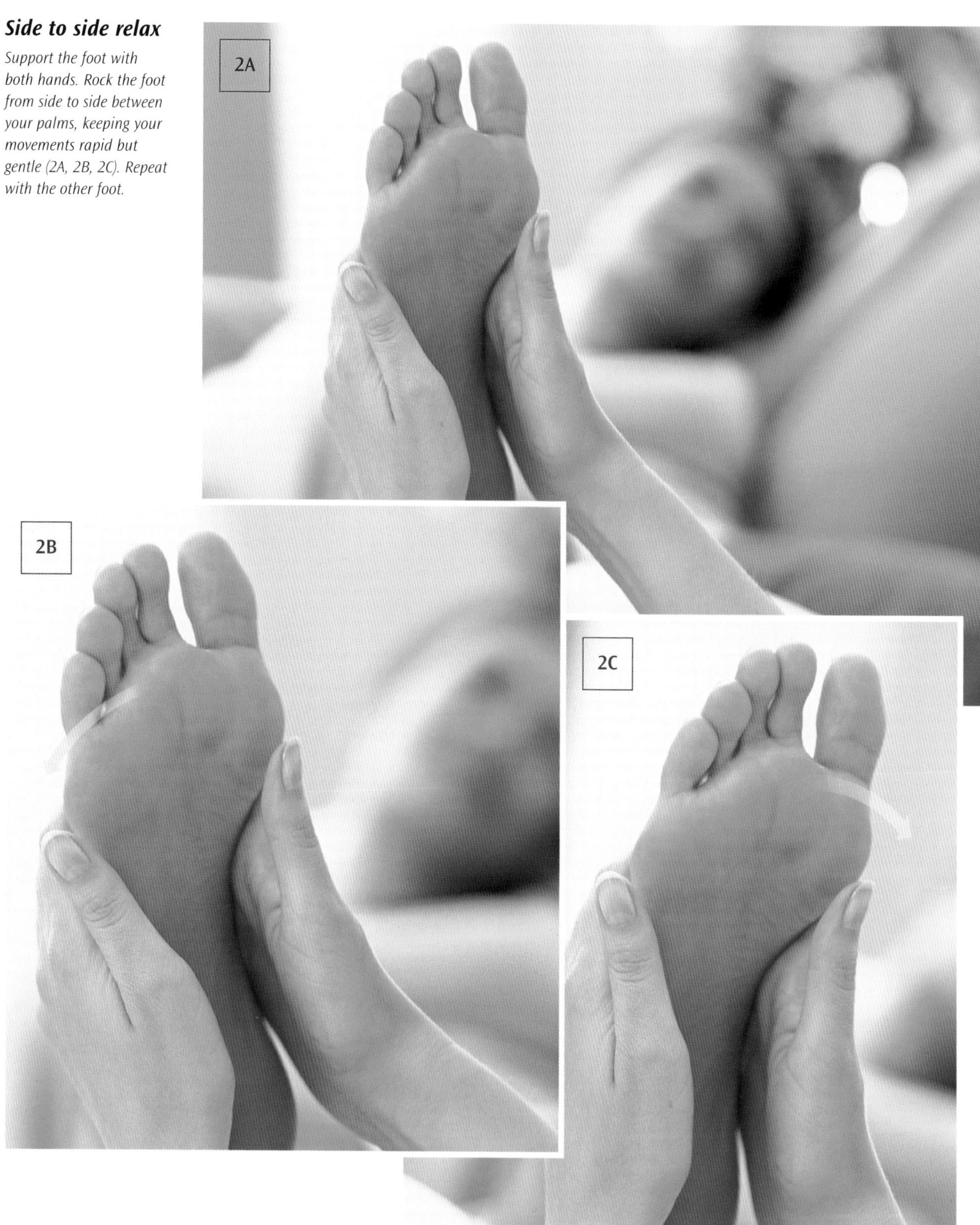

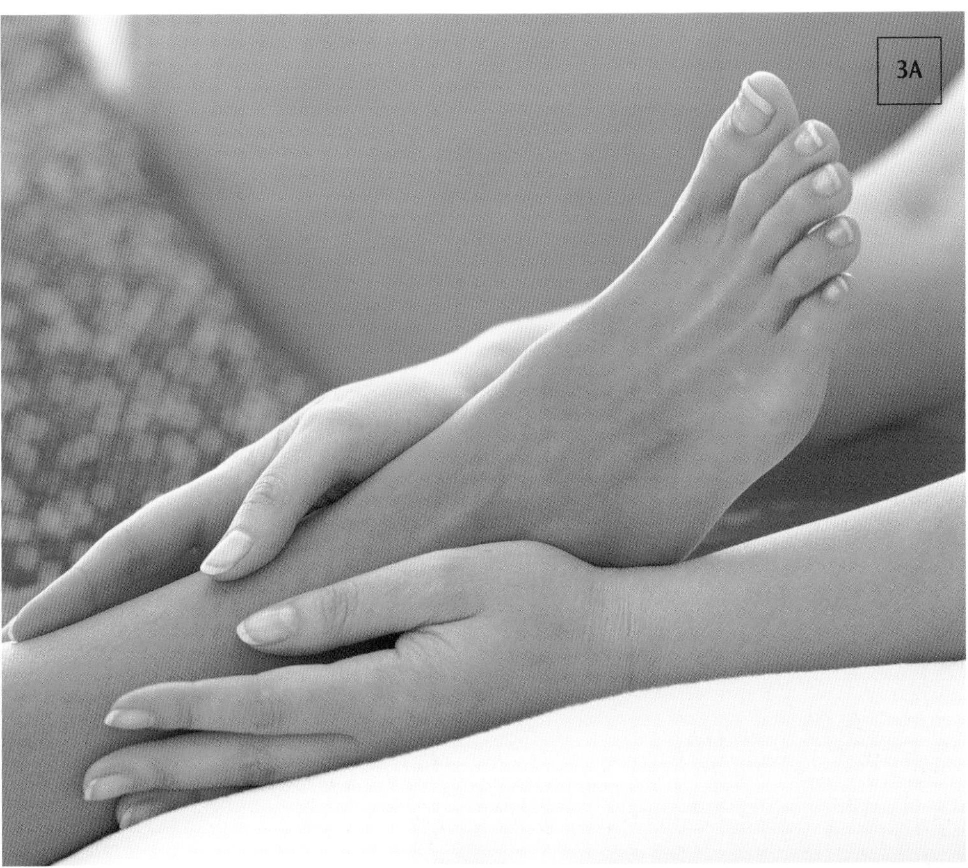

Ankle freeing

This is particularly helpful for anyone suffering from arthritis in the feet. Place your hands around the ankle, with the fleshy parts of your thumbs supporting the ankle bones. Gently but rapidly rock the foot from side to side, keeping your wrists loose. Keep your movements gentle and don't force the foot to move from side to side (3A, 3B).

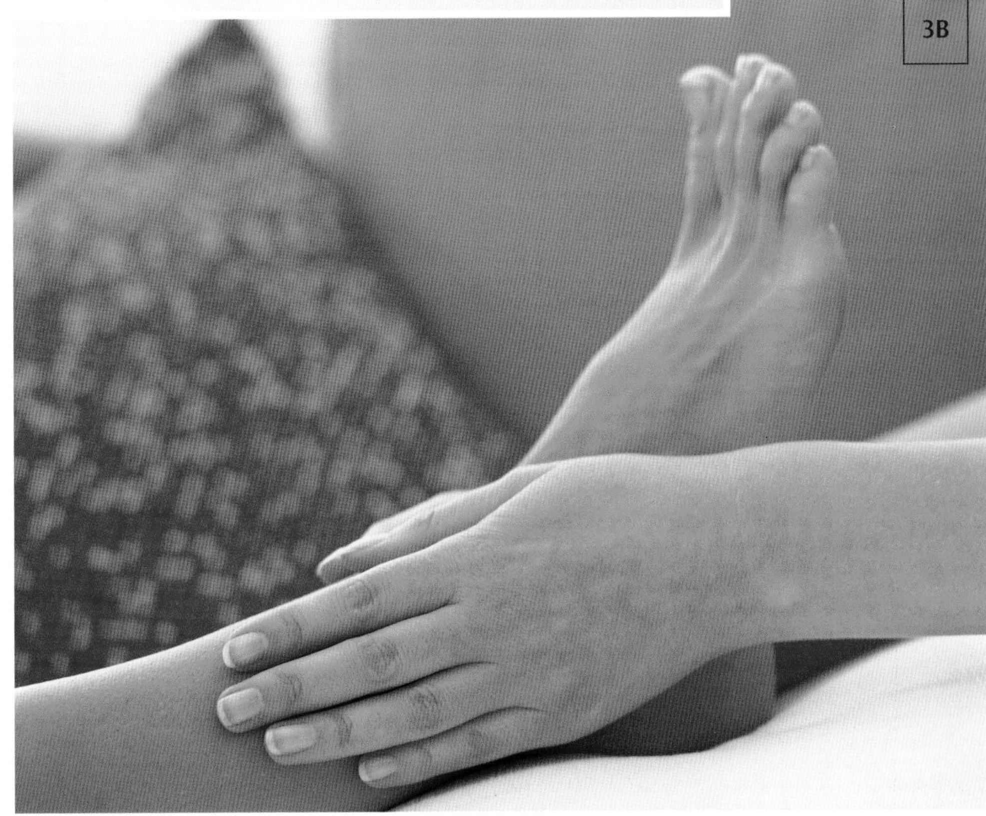

Metatarsal kneading

Start with the right foot. Make a fist with your right hand and push into the sole of the foot. At the same time, squeeze the top of the foot with your left hand as if you're kneading dough. Switch hands to treat the left foot (4).

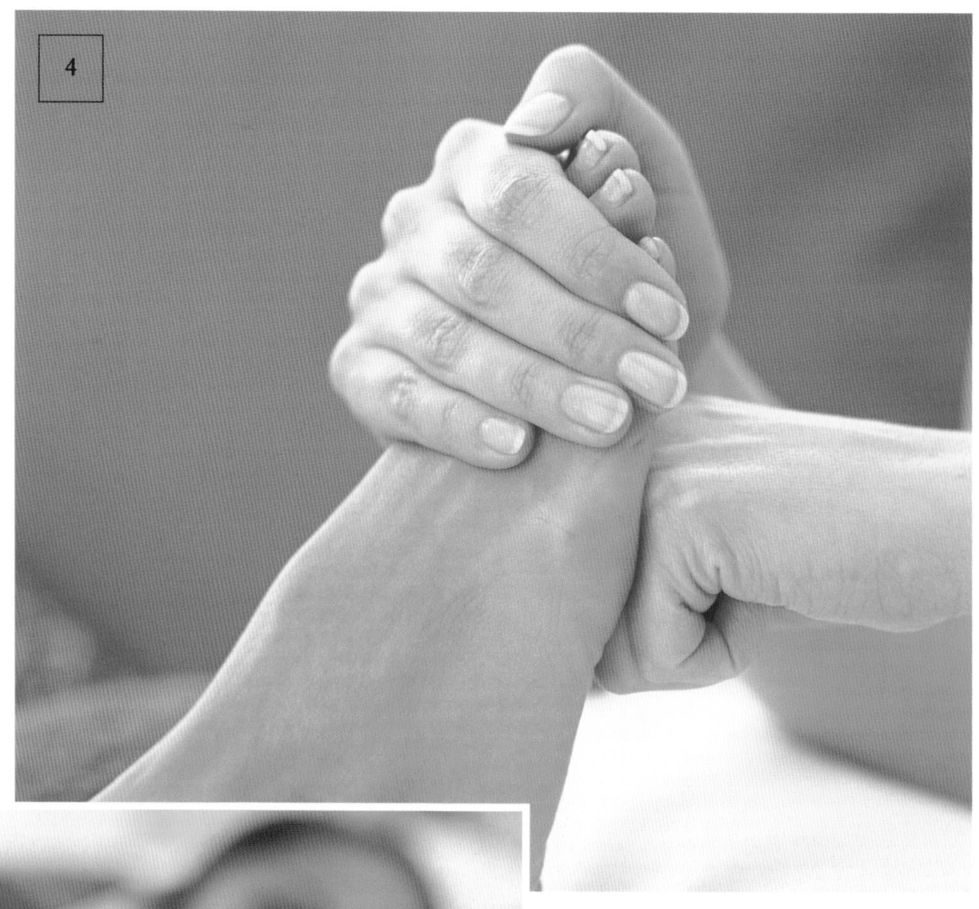

Energizing point one

This is the vital contact point for the whole of the central nervous system and vertebral column. You'll find it at the narrowest part of the foot on the medial side. Support the foot with your left hand and using your right thumb, press down on this point. Use a rotating movement in toward the spine (see page 20) to a count of five, pause and repeat (5).

Spinal friction

This stimulates and warms up the whole spinal column. Using the flat of your hand, rub vigorously up and down the medial (inside) edge of each foot (6).

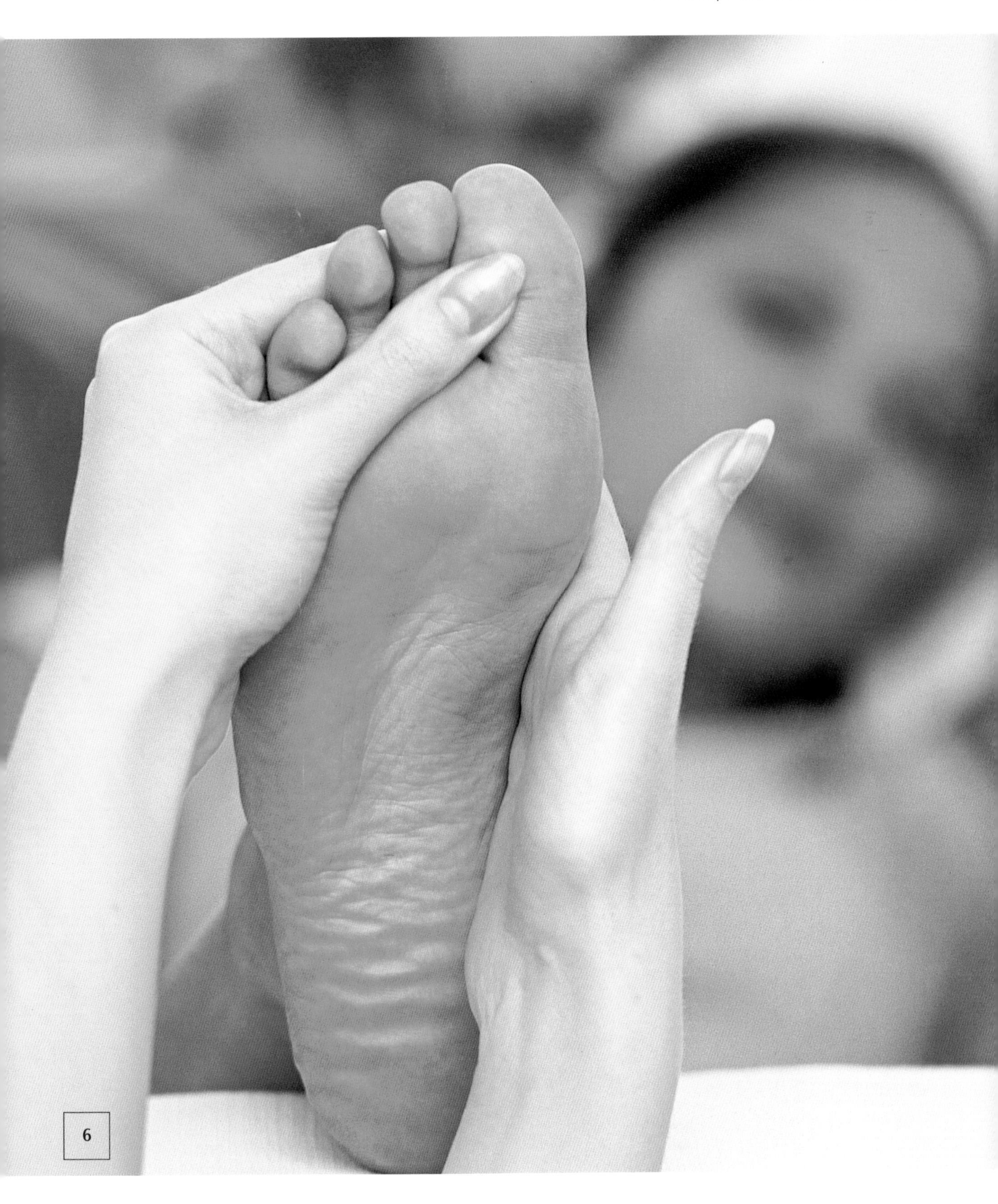

6

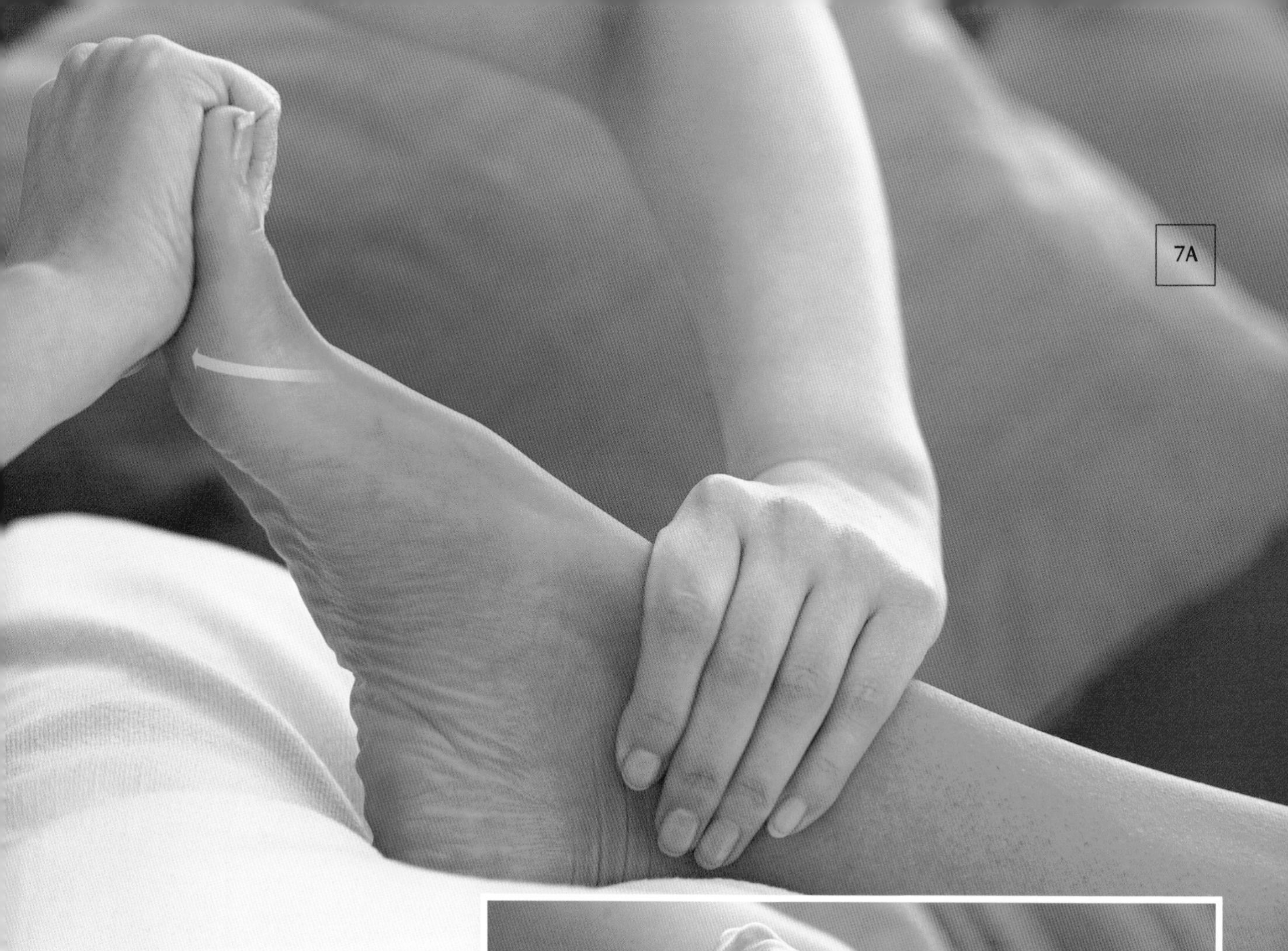

Circling (overgrip)

This relaxation exercise helps to soothe swollen ankles and reduce swelling. Starting with the right foot, place your left hand around the top of the ankle, making sure that your thumb is on the lateral edge of the foot (7A). Using your right hand, circle the foot inward and toward the spine (7B). For the left foot, hold the ankle with your right hand and circle with your left.

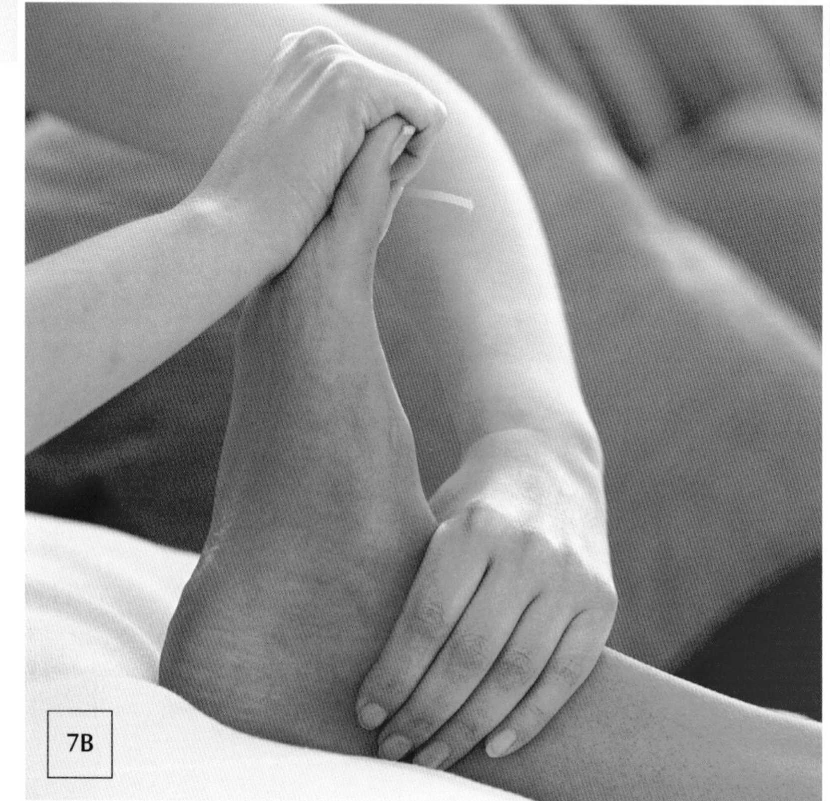

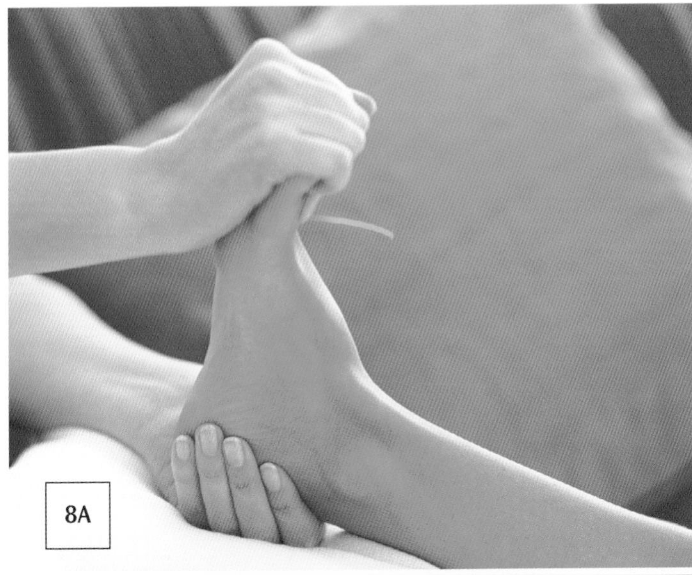

Circling (undergrip)

Support the heel of the right foot with your left hand (8A). With your right hand, gently circle the foot inward and toward the spine (8B). Repeat on the left foot, supporting the foot with your right hand and circling with your left.

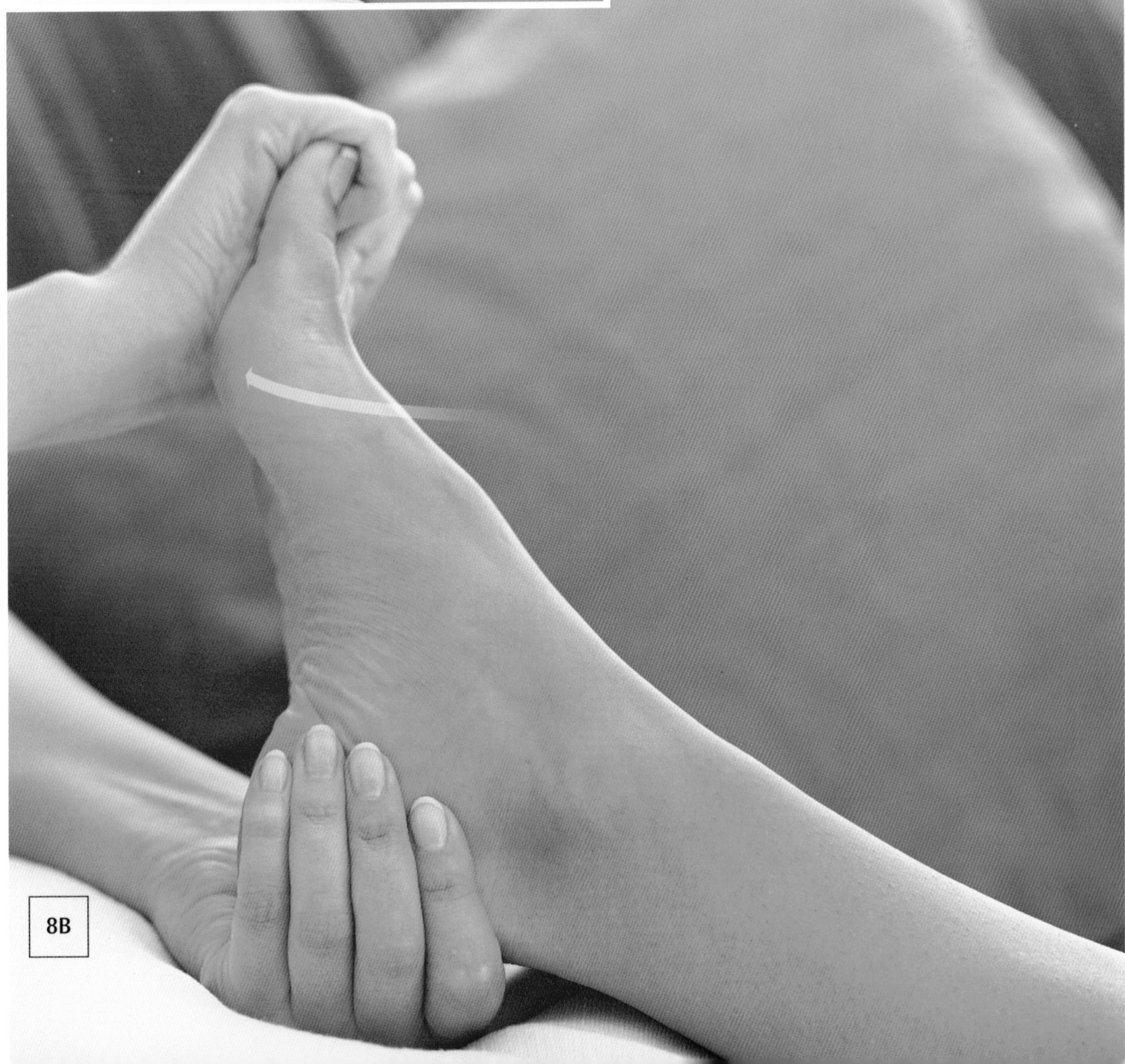

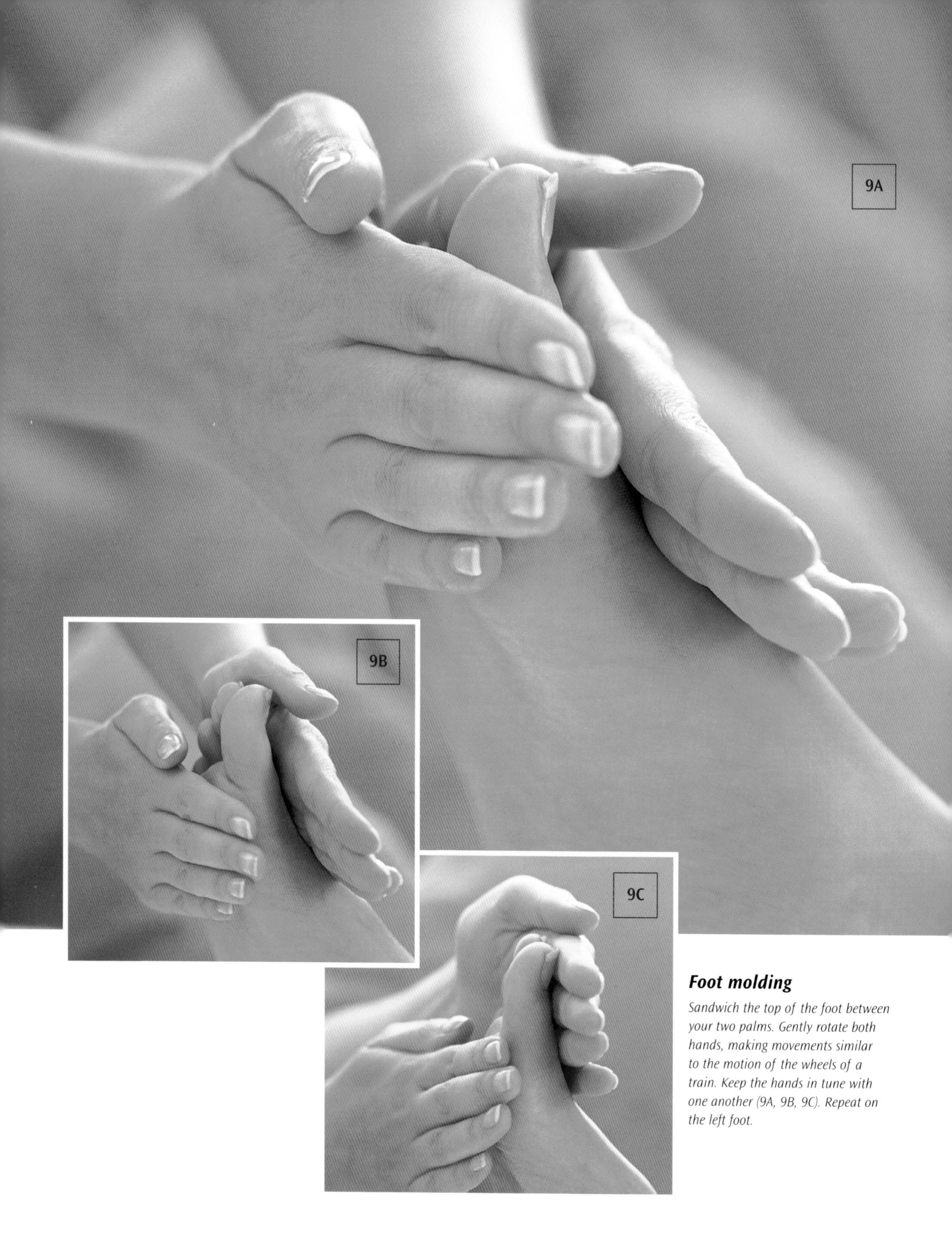

Foot molding

Sandwich the top of the foot between your two palms. Gently rotate both hands, making movements similar to the motion of the wheels of a train. Keep the hands in tune with one another (9A, 9B, 9C). Repeat on the left foot.

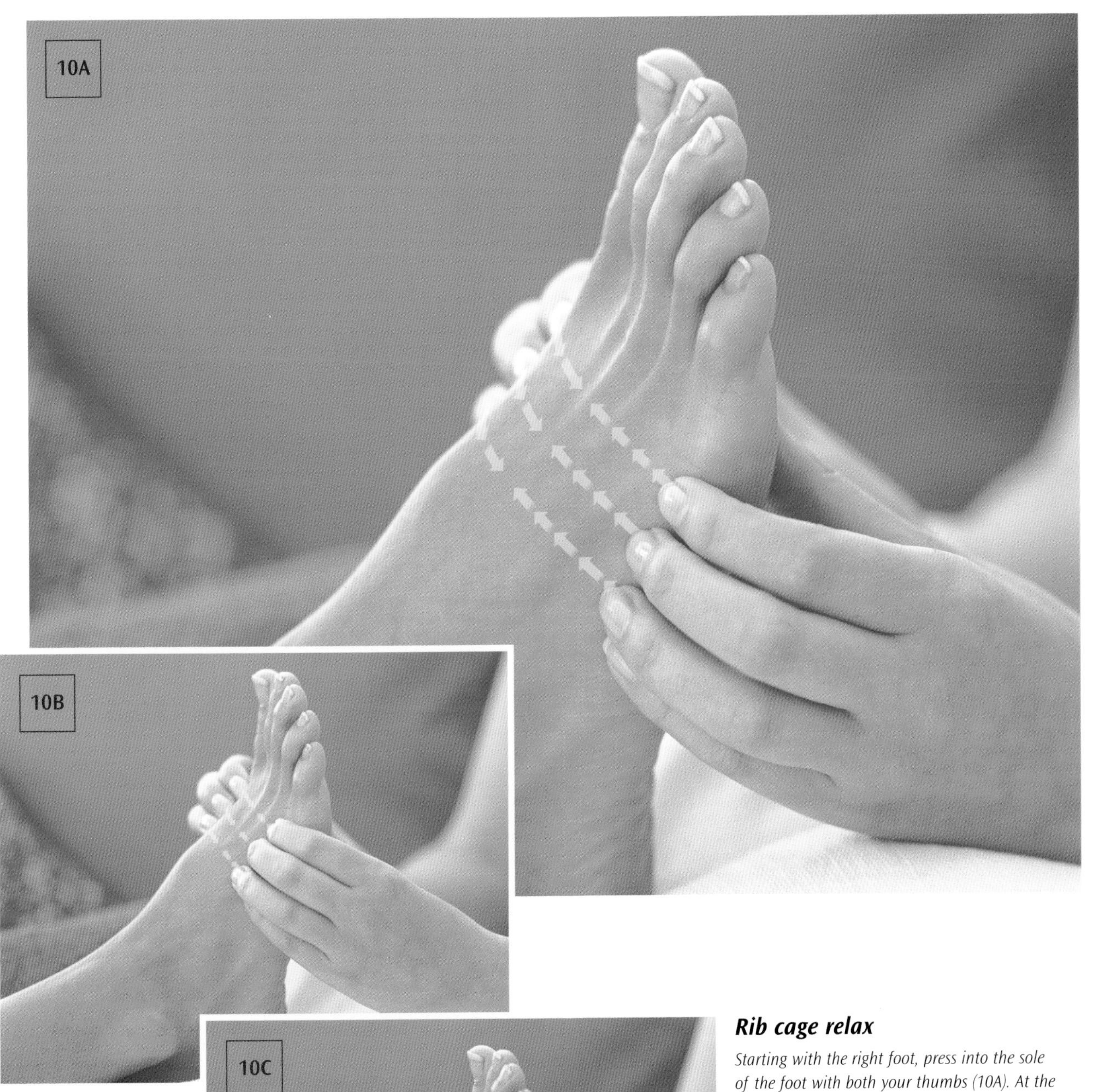

Rib cage relax

Starting with the right foot, press into the sole of the foot with both your thumbs (10A). At the same time, creep across the top of the foot with the fingers of both hands. Work toward the middle as shown (10B, 10C). Repeat on the left foot.

Once the feet are relaxed, start the treatment session on all areas of the body.

Breast and lung (plantar)

Support the right foot with your left hand. Using your thumb, creep up the areas between the grooves of each toe (11) on the plantar side of the foot. Switch hands to work the left foot.

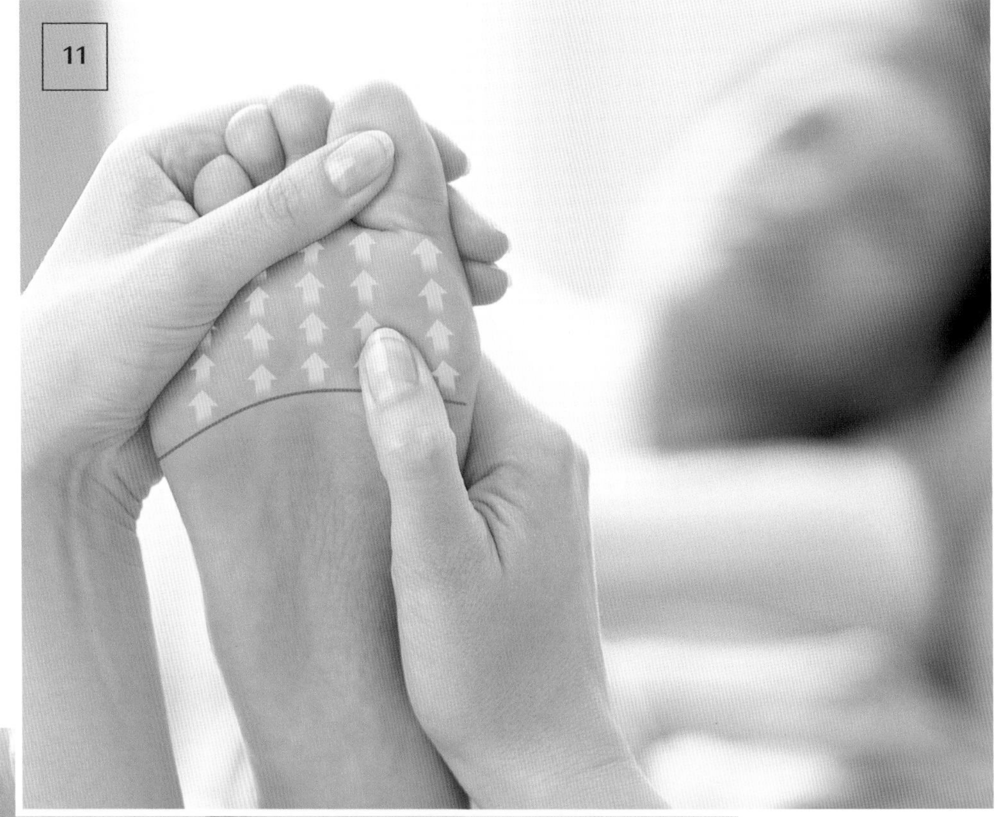
11

12

Breast and lung (dorsal)

Make a fist with your left hand and press it into the sole of the right foot. Using your right index finger, creep down the grooves below the toes on the top of the foot (12). Switch hands to work the left foot.

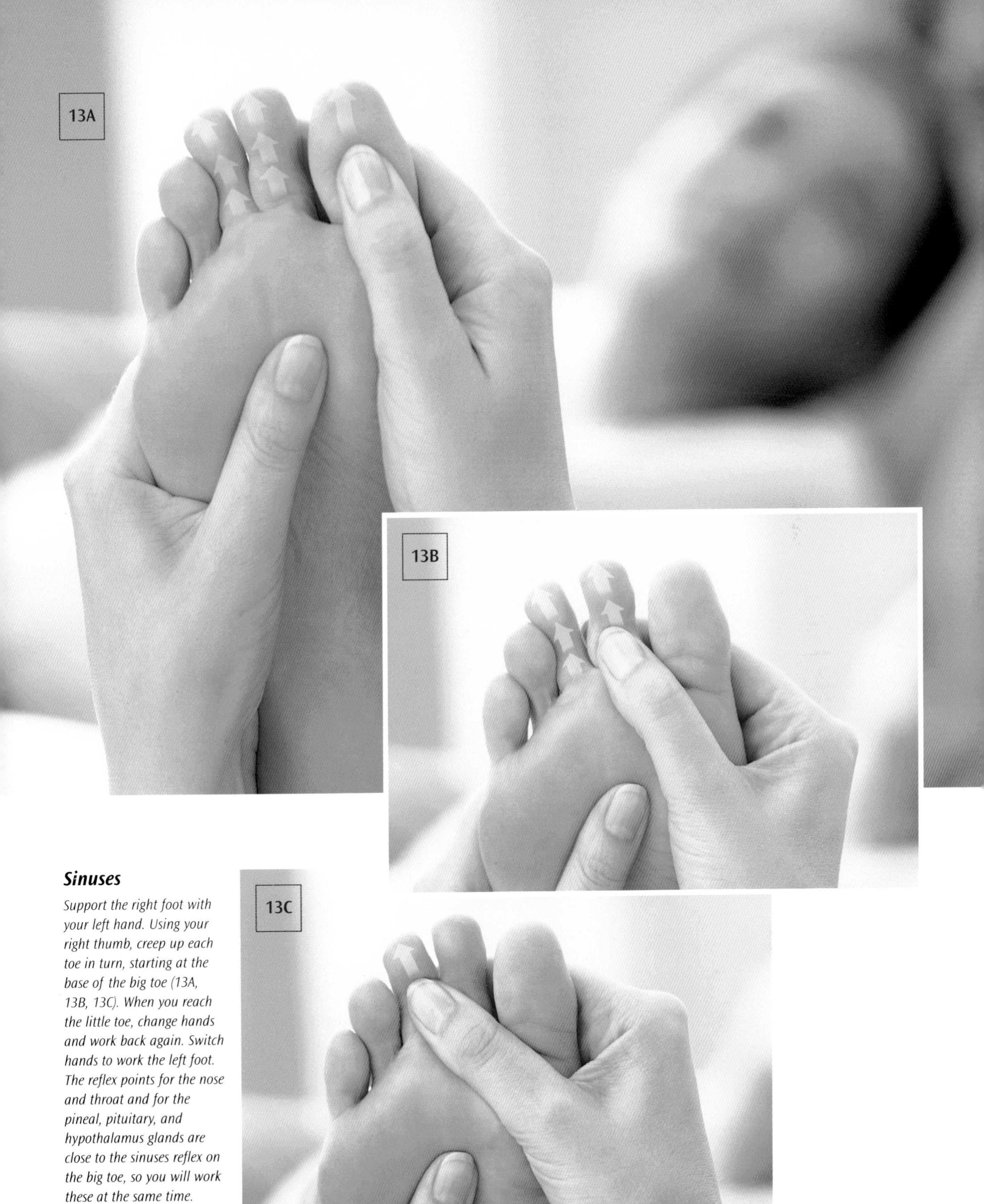

Sinuses

Support the right foot with your left hand. Using your right thumb, creep up each toe in turn, starting at the base of the big toe (13A, 13B, 13C). When you reach the little toe, change hands and work back again. Switch hands to work the left foot. The reflex points for the nose and throat and for the pineal, pituitary, and hypothalamus glands are close to the sinuses reflex on the big toe, so you will work these at the same time.

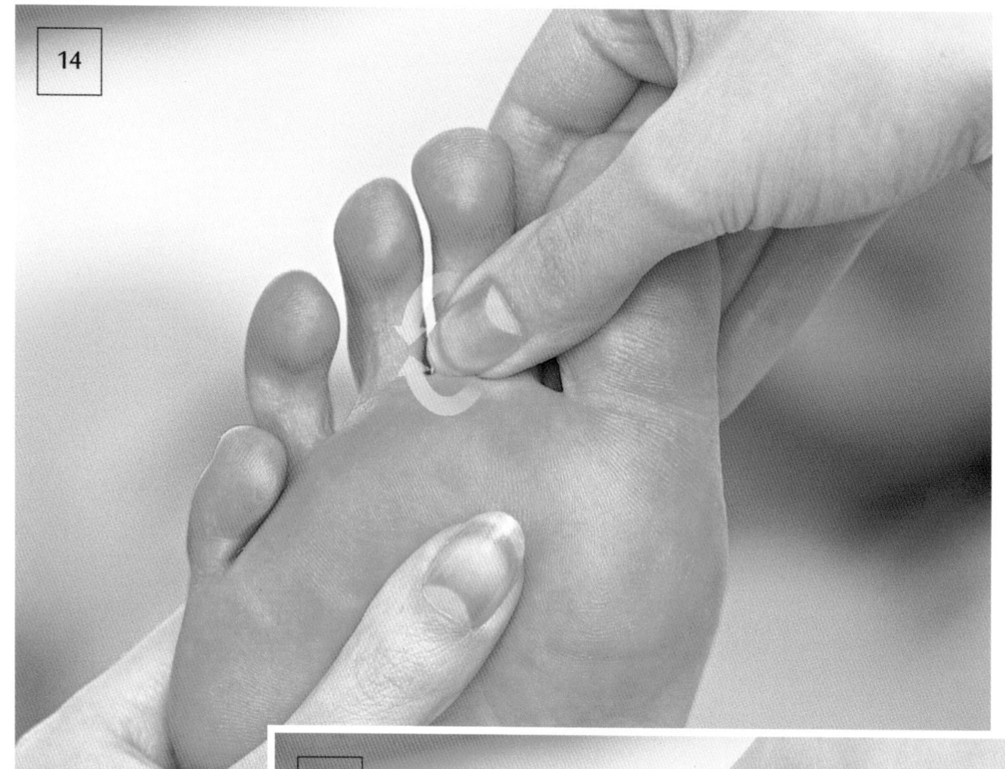

Eye

Support the right foot with your left hand. Place your right thumb just under the first bend of the second toe and work the reflex with a small clockwise rotating movement (14). Switch hands to work the left foot.

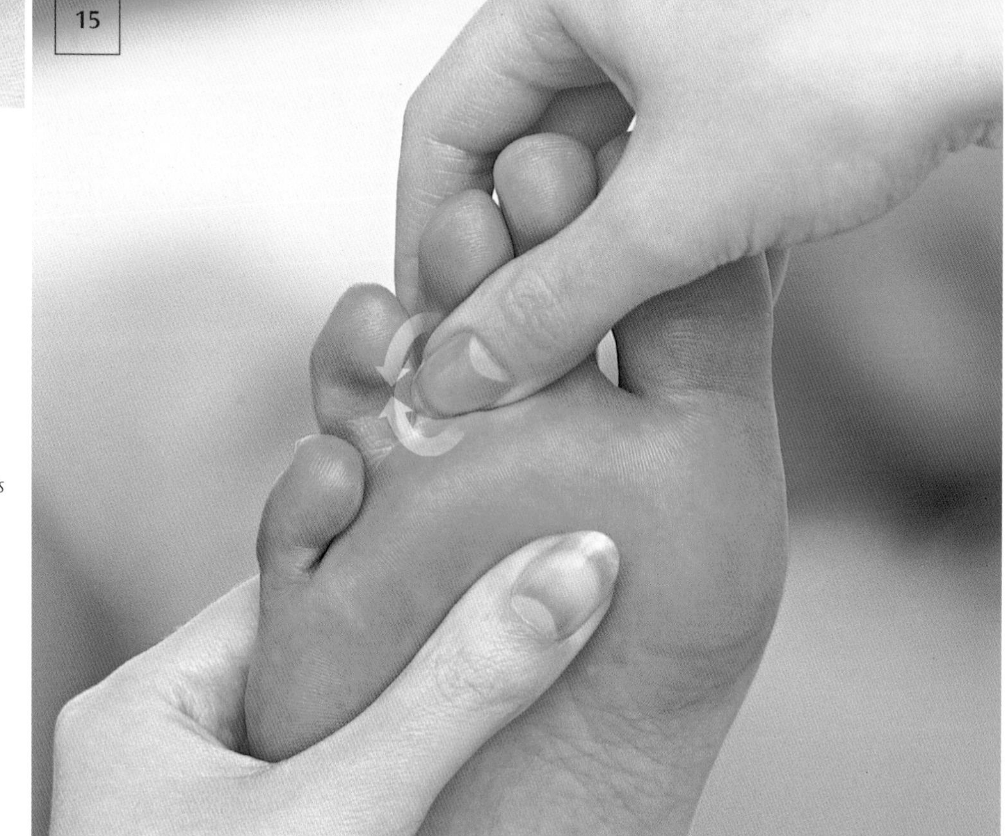

Ear

Support the right foot with your left hand. Place your right thumb just under the first bend of the third toe and work the reflex with a small clockwise rotating movement (15). Switch hands to work the left foot.

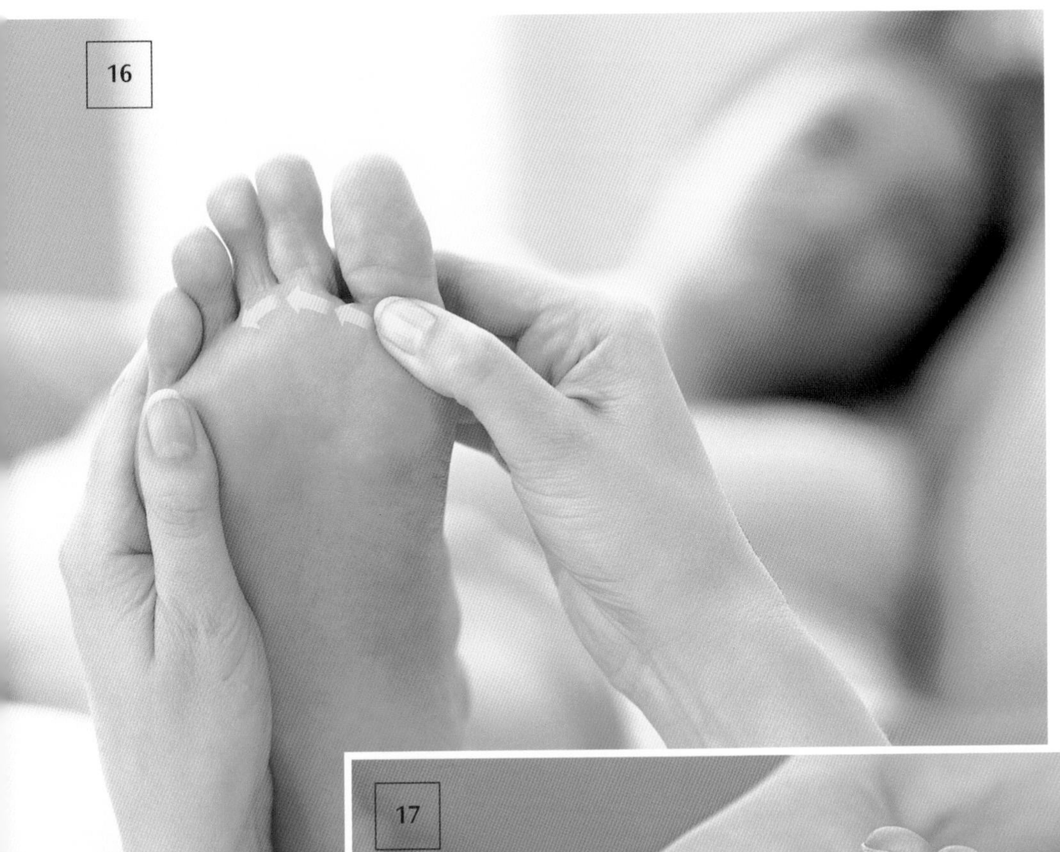

Neck and thyroid (plantar)

Support the right foot with your left hand. Using your right thumb, creep across the bases of the first three toes (16). Repeat three times. Switch hands to work the left foot.

Neck and thyroid (dorsal)

Support the right foot against your left fist. Using your right index finger, creep along the bases of the first three toes (17). Repeat three times. Switch hands to work the left foot.

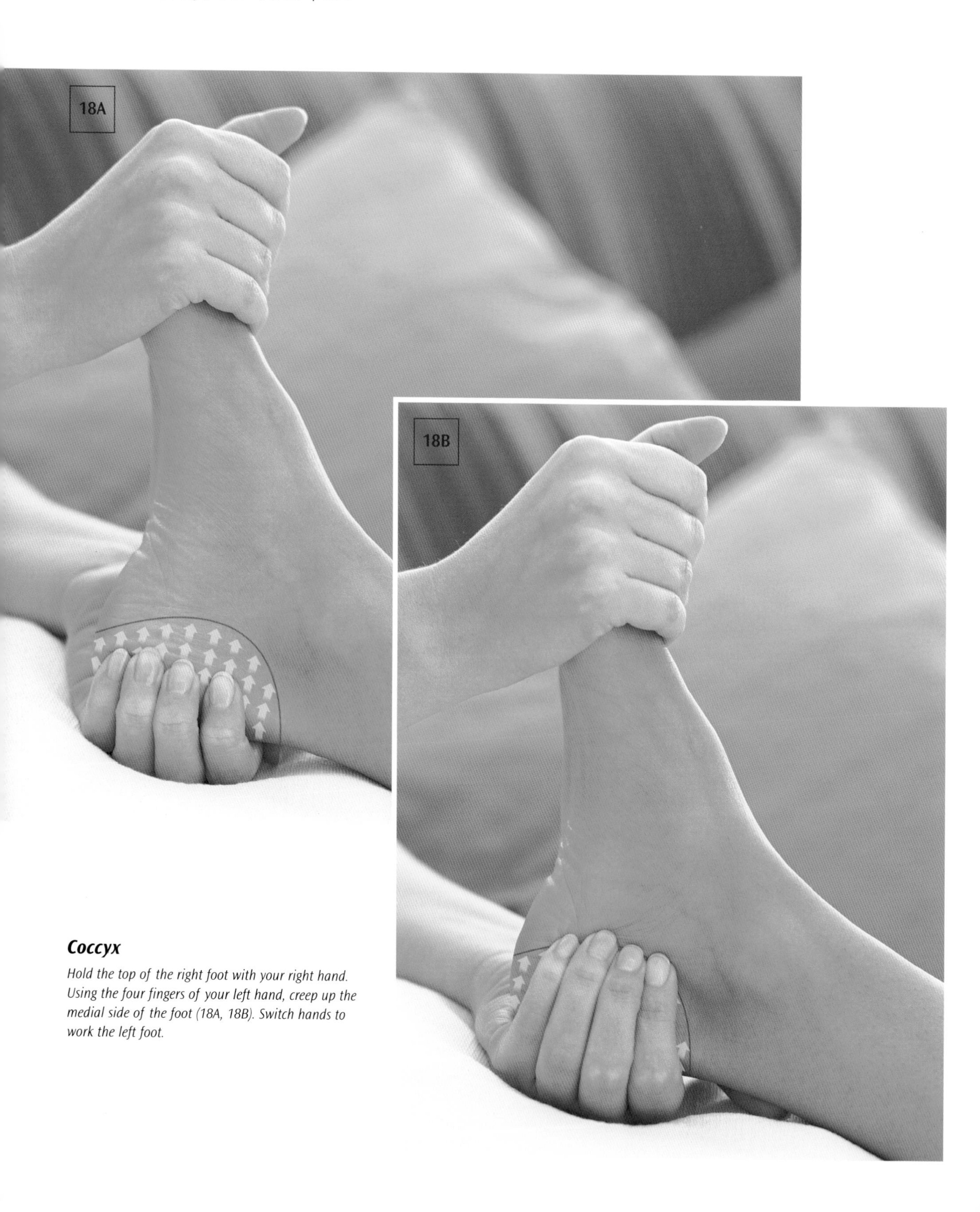

Coccyx

Hold the top of the right foot with your right hand. Using the four fingers of your left hand, creep up the medial side of the foot (18A, 18B). Switch hands to work the left foot.

Hip and pelvis

Support the top of the right foot with your left hand. Using the four fingers of your right hand, creep up the lateral side of the heel (19A, 19B). Switch hands to work the left foot.

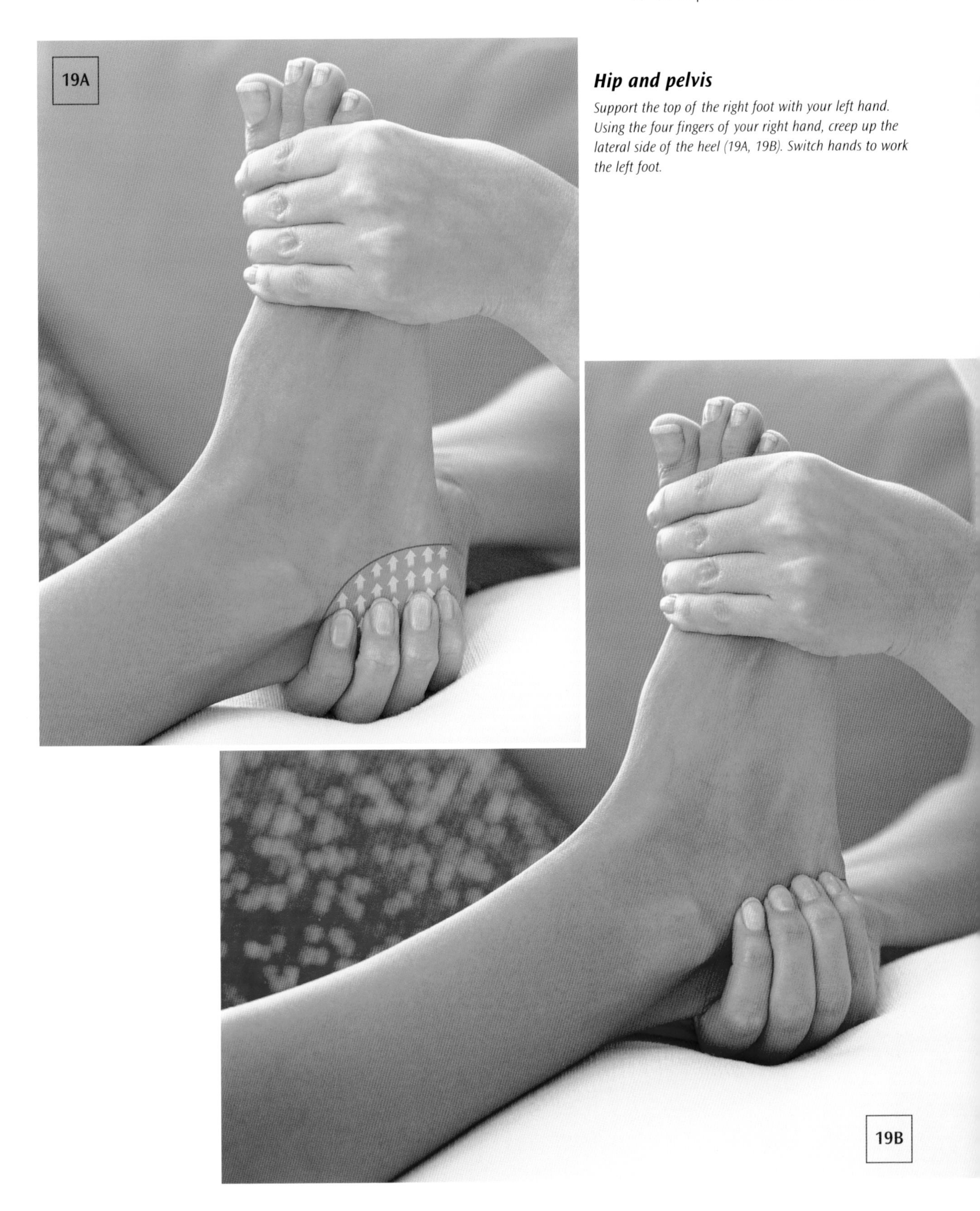

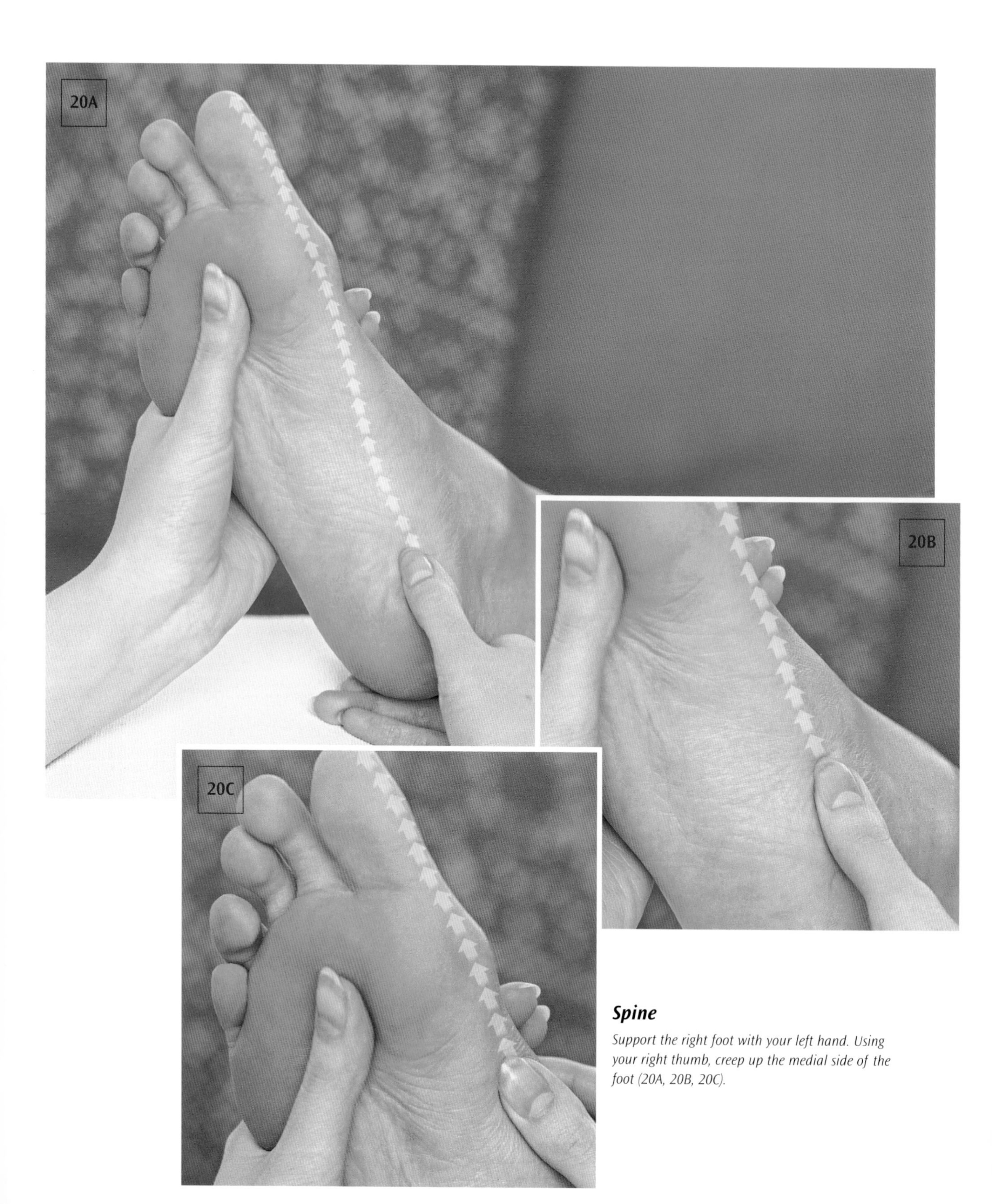

Spine

Support the right foot with your left hand. Using your right thumb, creep up the medial side of the foot (20A, 20B, 20C).

Spine

Continue creeping up the medial side of the foot to the big toe (20D, 20E). Switch hands to work the left foot.

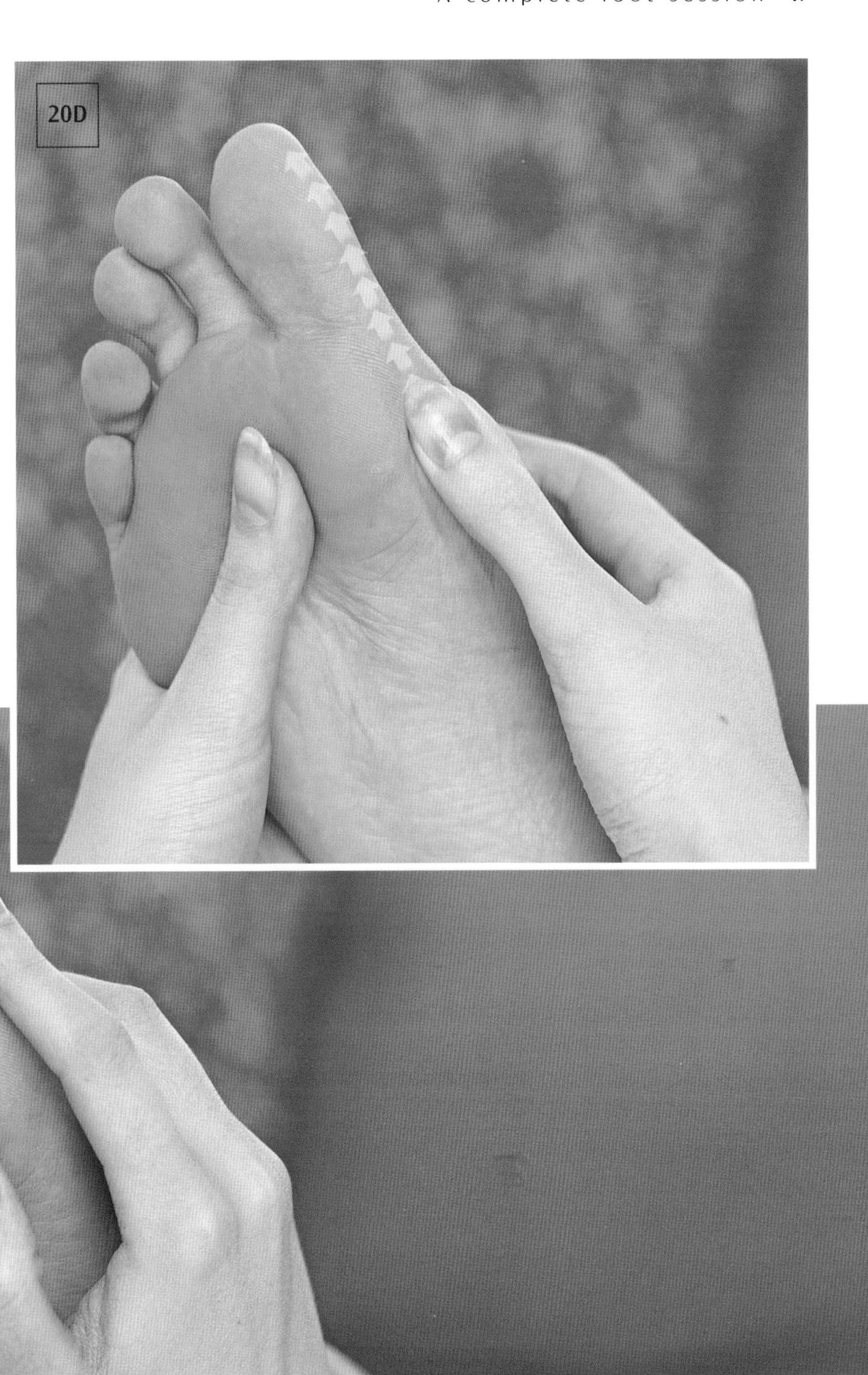

Chronic neck conditions

Support the right foot with your left hand. Using your right thumb, work down the lateral sides of the first three toes (21A, 21B, 21C). Switch hands to work the left foot.

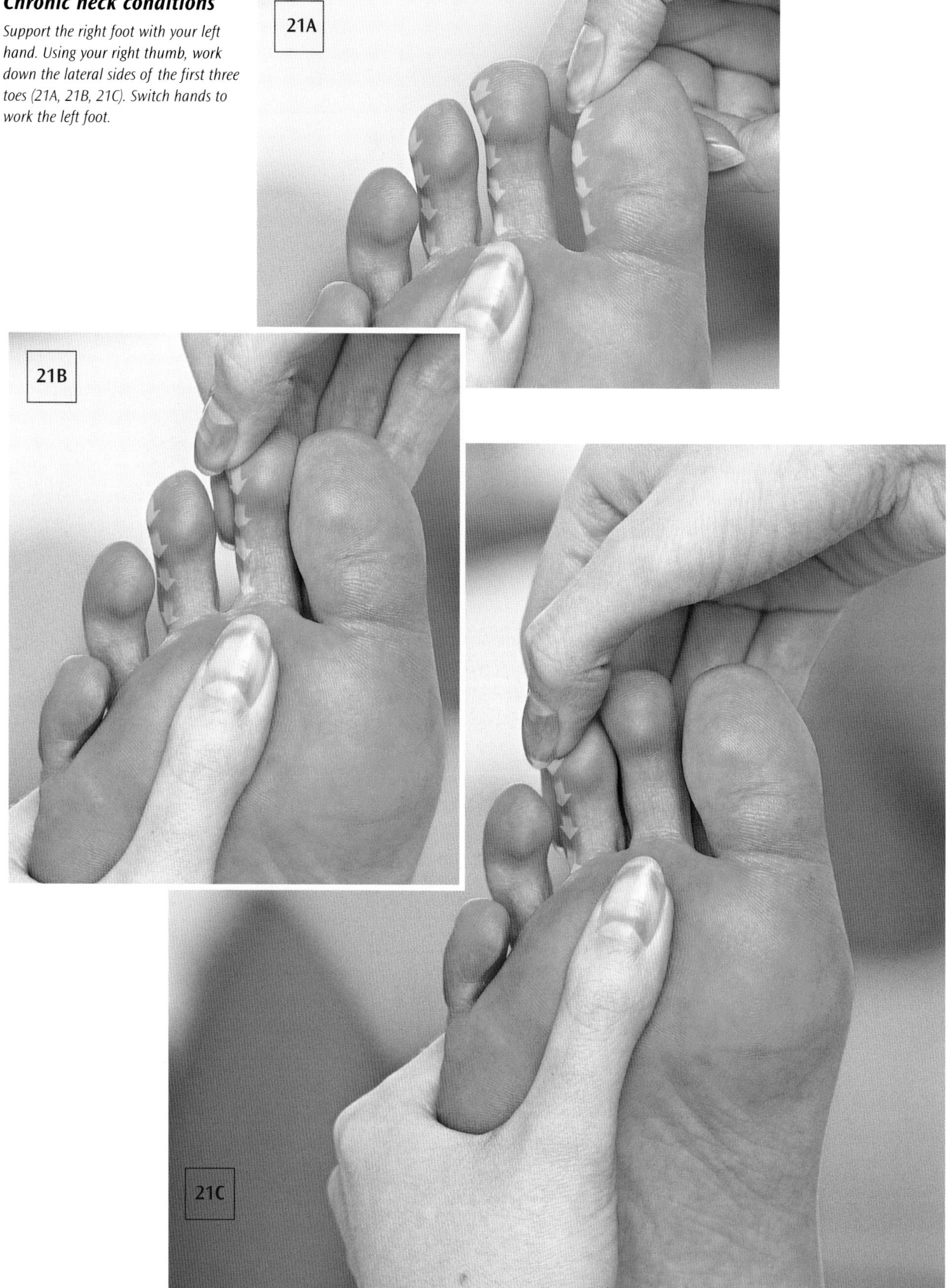

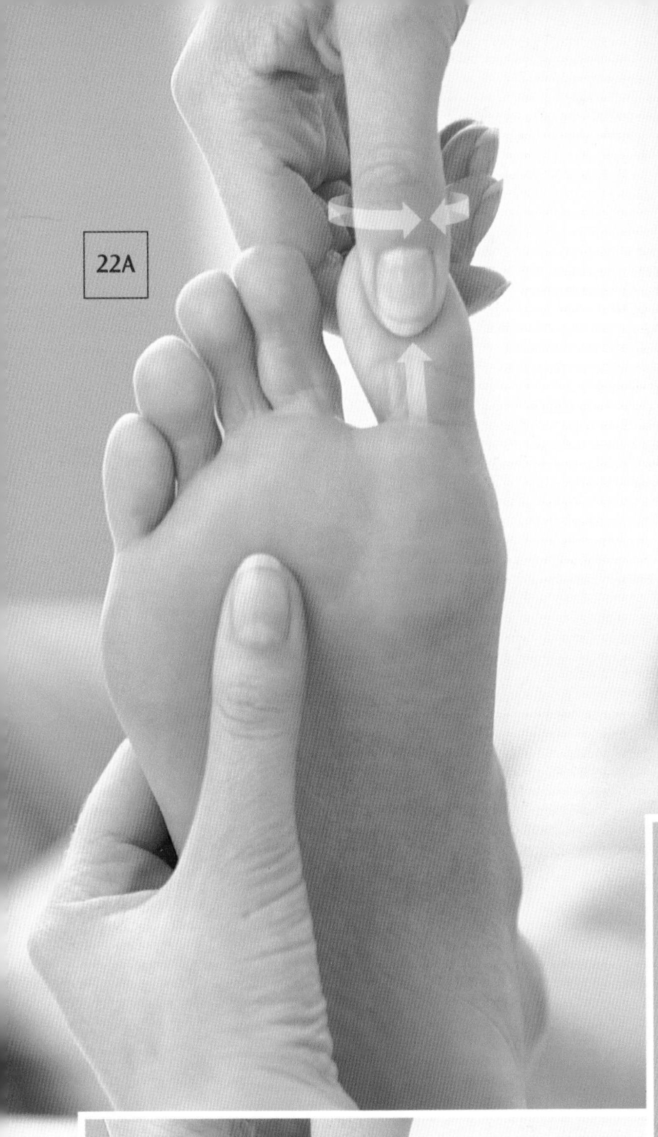

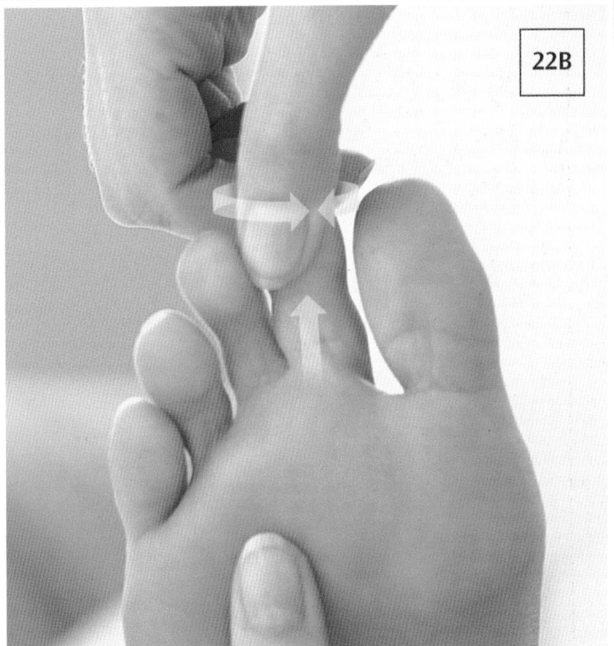

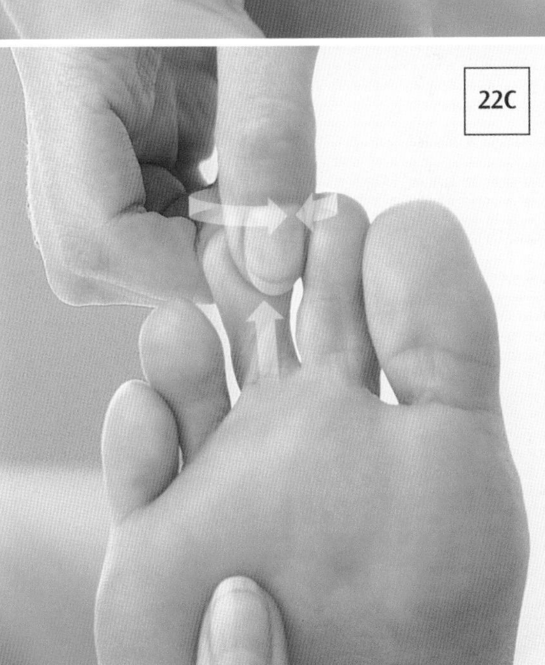

Neck rotation

Support the right foot with your left hand. Using your right thumb, lift and rotate each of the first three toes in turn (22A, 22B, 22C). Switch hands to work the left foot. This is particularly helpful for stiff necks.

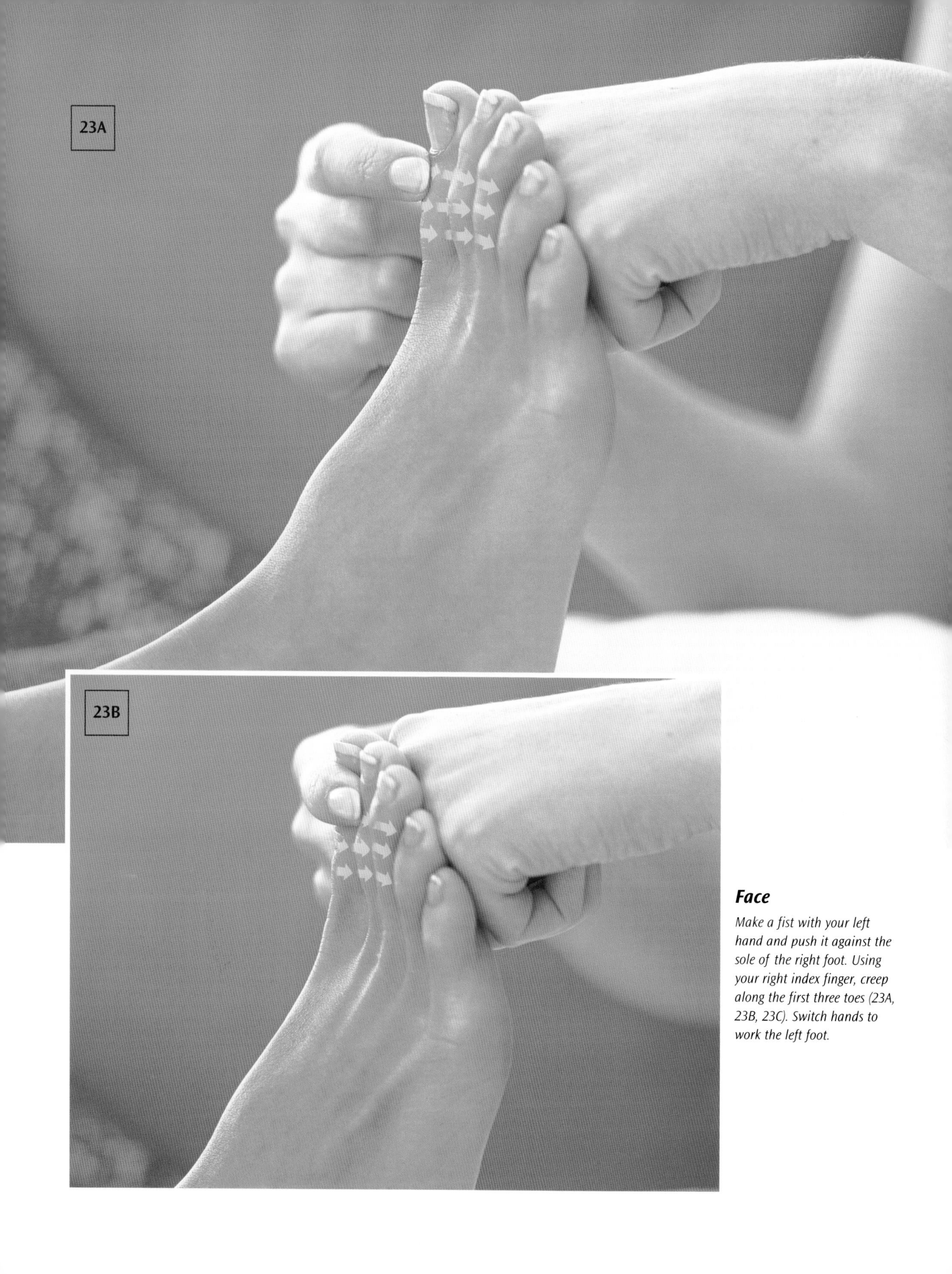

Face

Make a fist with your left hand and push it against the sole of the right foot. Using your right index finger, creep along the first three toes (23A, 23B, 23C). Switch hands to work the left foot.

23C

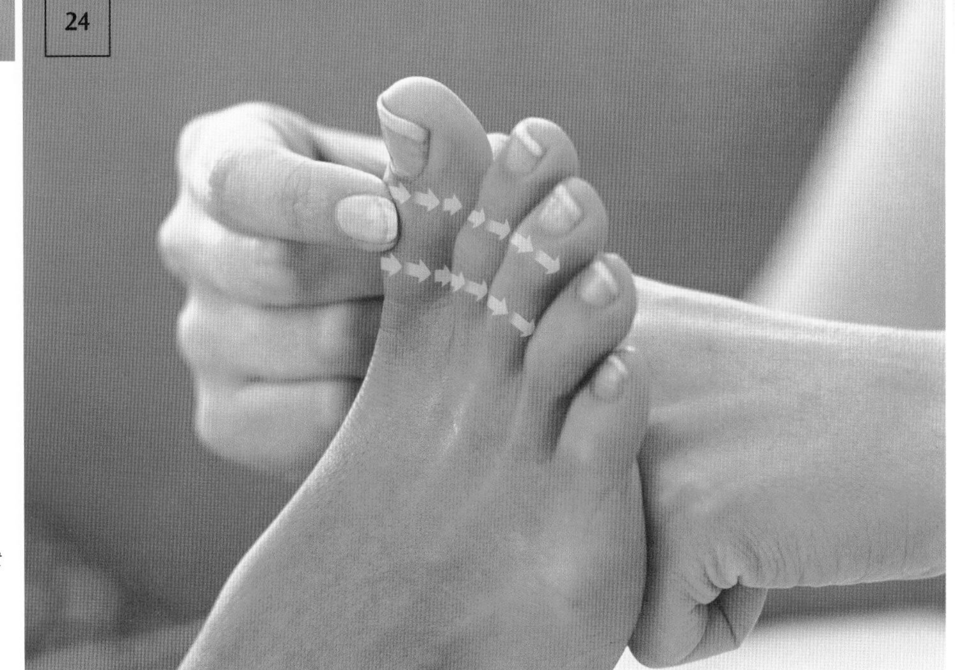

Teeth

This treatment helps to relieve tooth pain while you're waiting to see your dentist or after having dentistry. Support the right foot against your left fist. For the upper jaw, use your index finger to work across the first three toes in line with the bases of the nails (24). For the lower jaw, work along the first three toes about ¼ inch (0.5 cm) above where the toes join the feet. Switch hands to work the left foot.

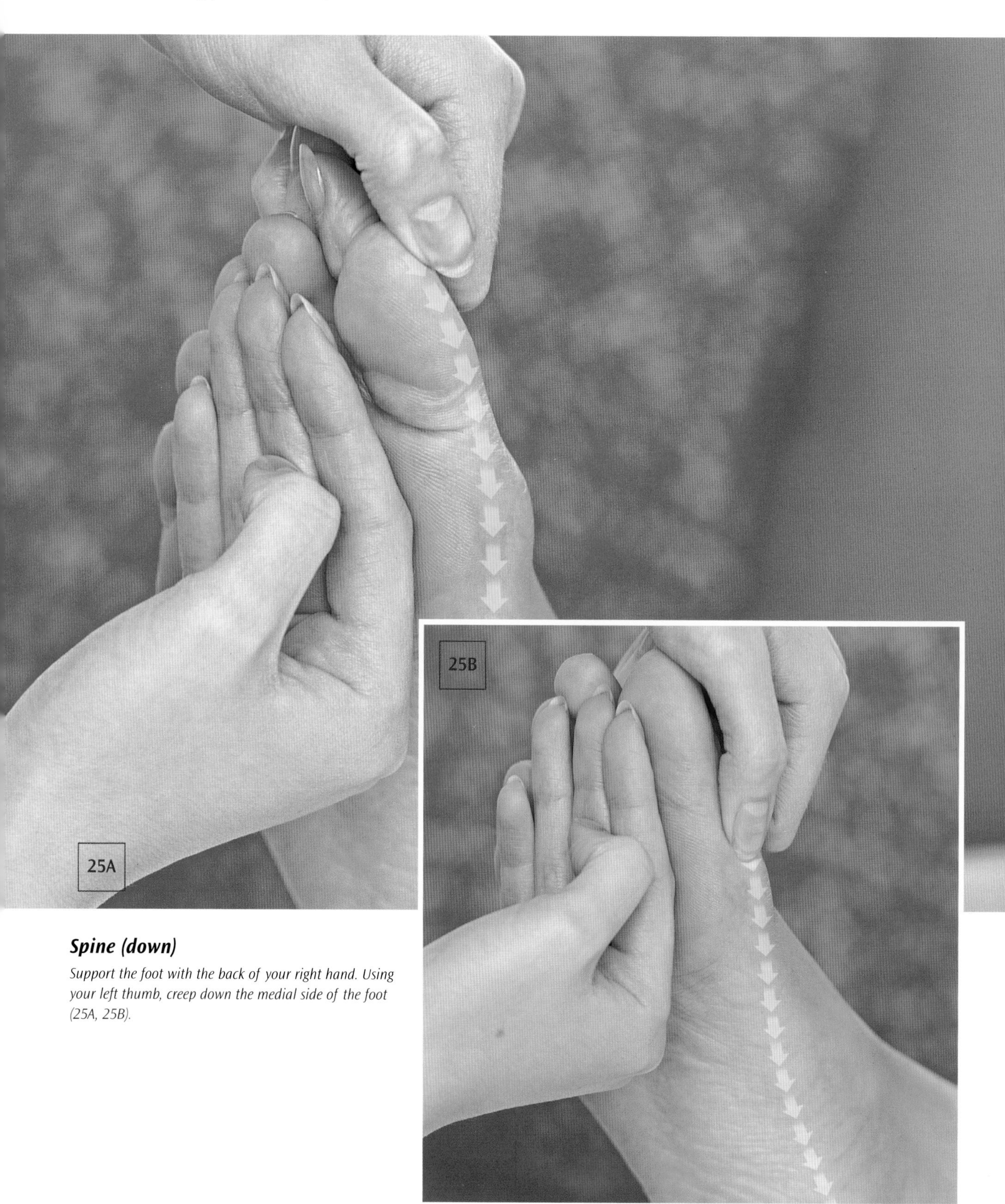

Spine (down)

Support the foot with the back of your right hand. Using your left thumb, creep down the medial side of the foot (25A, 25B).

Spine (down)

Continue working down the medial side of the foot, moving the supporting hand down as you go (25C). When you reach the heel area, support the foot with the back of your non-working hand (25D, 25E). Switch hands to work the left foot.

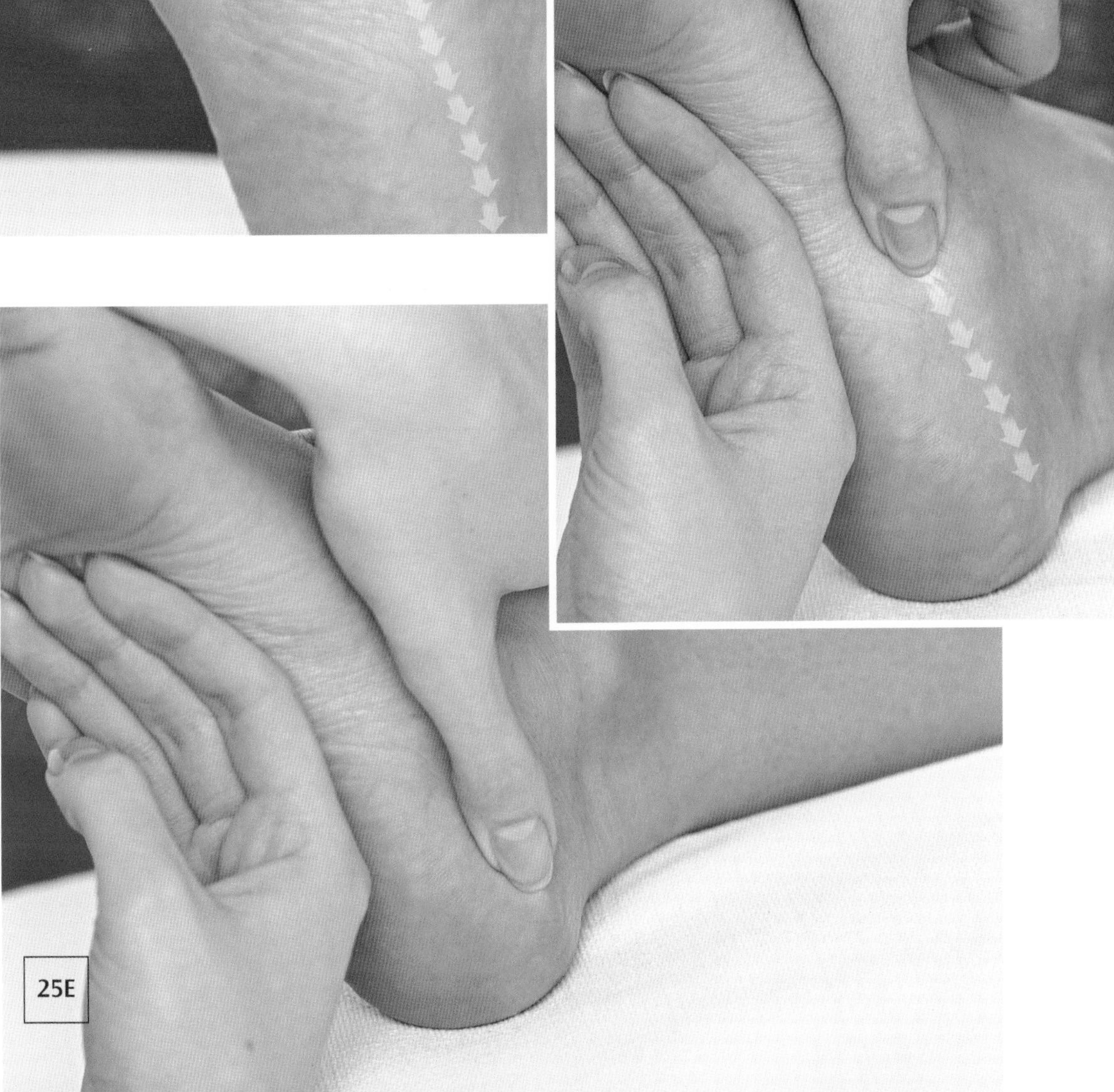

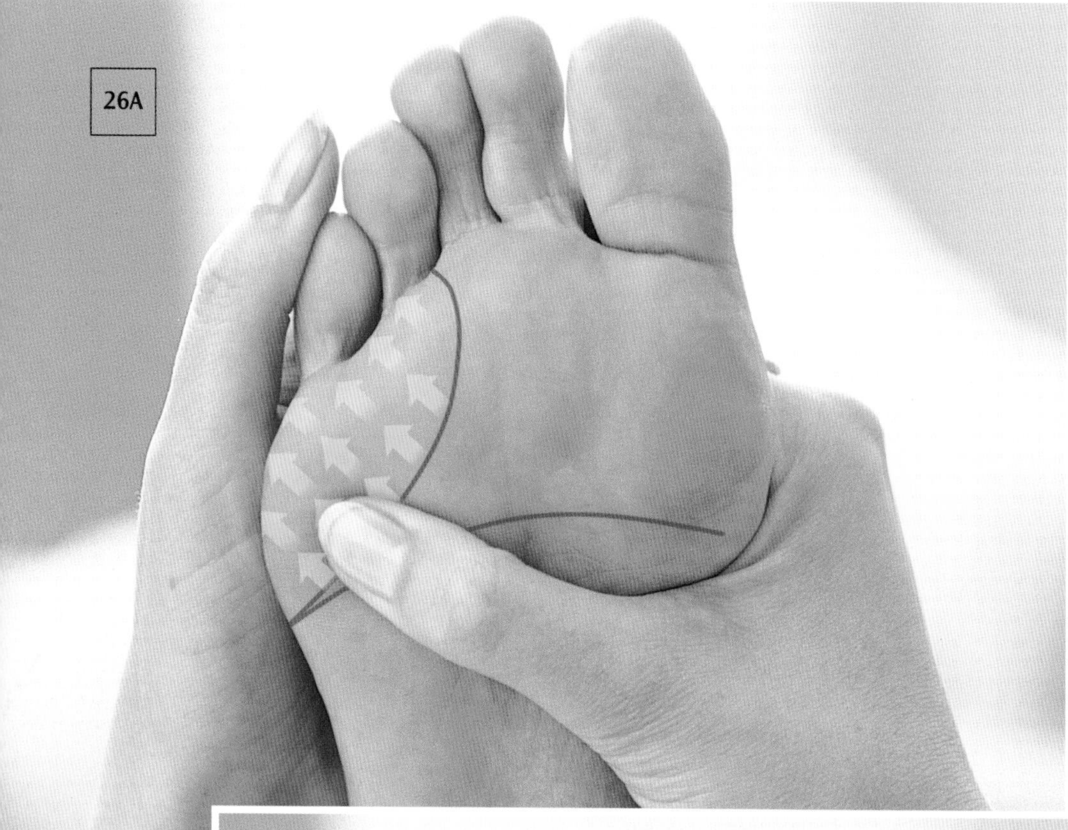

Shoulder (plantar)

Support the right foot with your left hand. Using your right thumb, creep outward across the shoulder reflex area (26A). Change hands and creep inward with your left thumb (26B). To work the left foot, start by supporting the foot with your right hand and creeping outward with your left thumb.

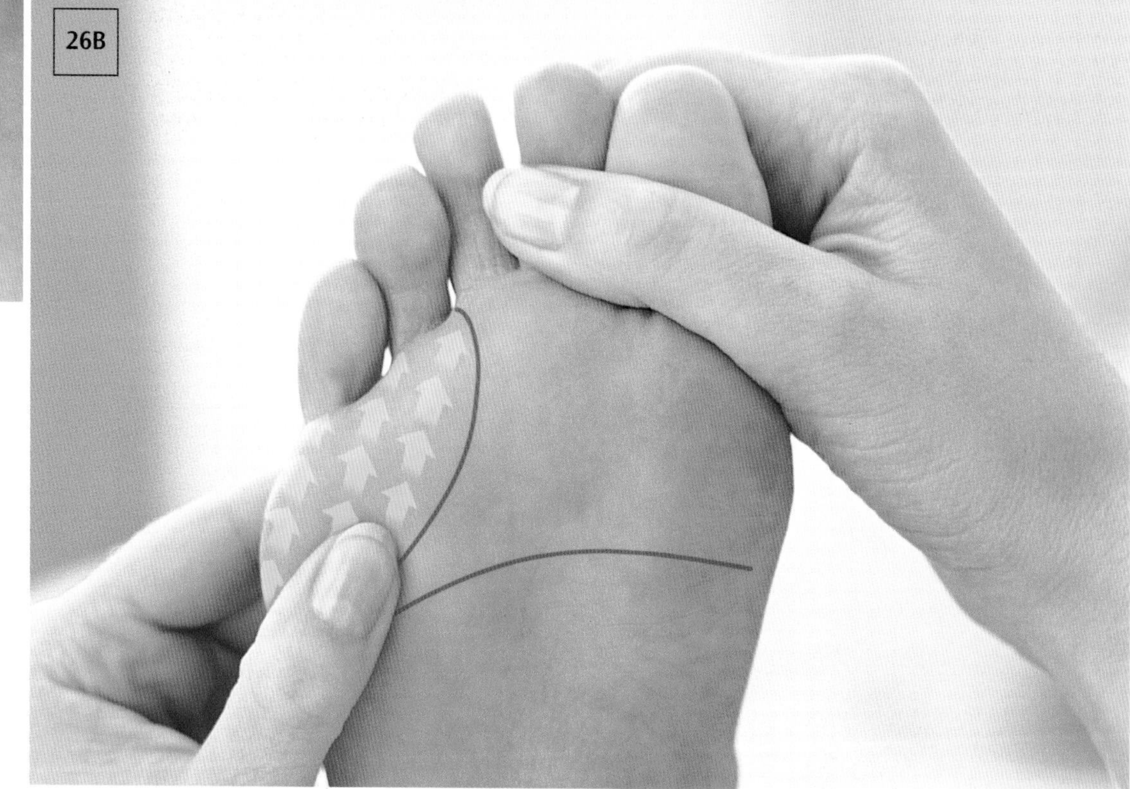

Shoulder (dorsal)

Support the right foot against your left fist. Using your right index finger, work down the grooves of the fourth and fifth toes (27A, 27B). Switch hands to work the left foot.

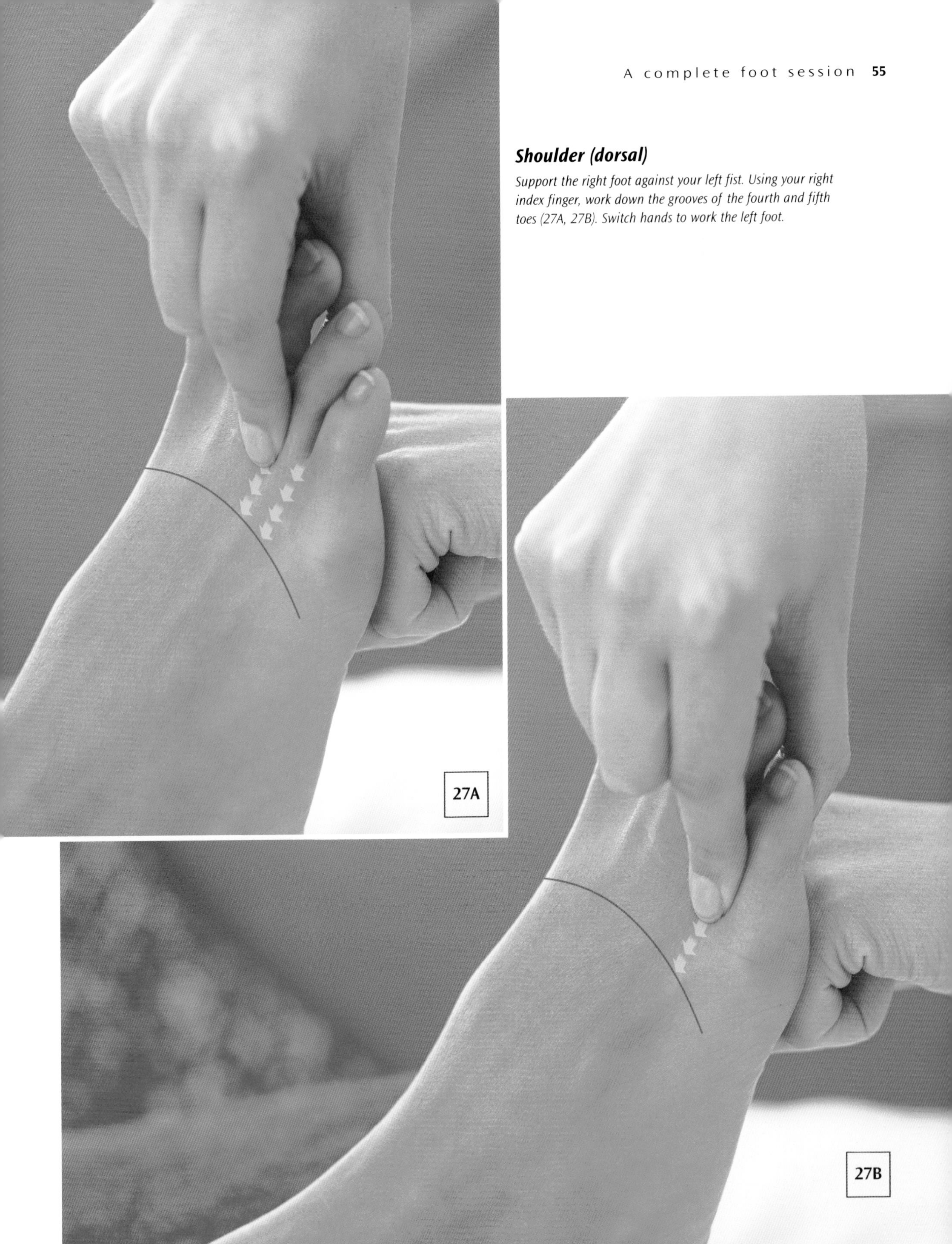

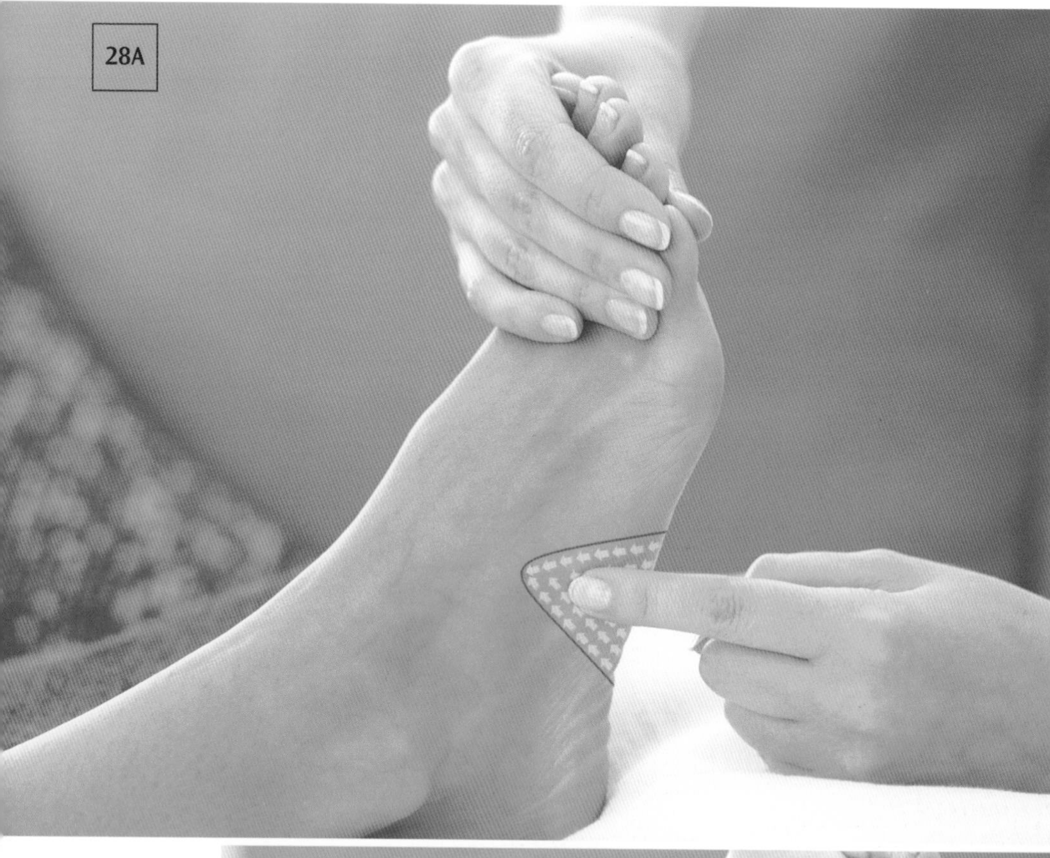

Knee and elbow

Support the right foot with your right hand. Using your left index finger, creep up the triangular-shaped reflex area on the lateral side of the foot (28A, 28B). Switch hands to work the left foot.

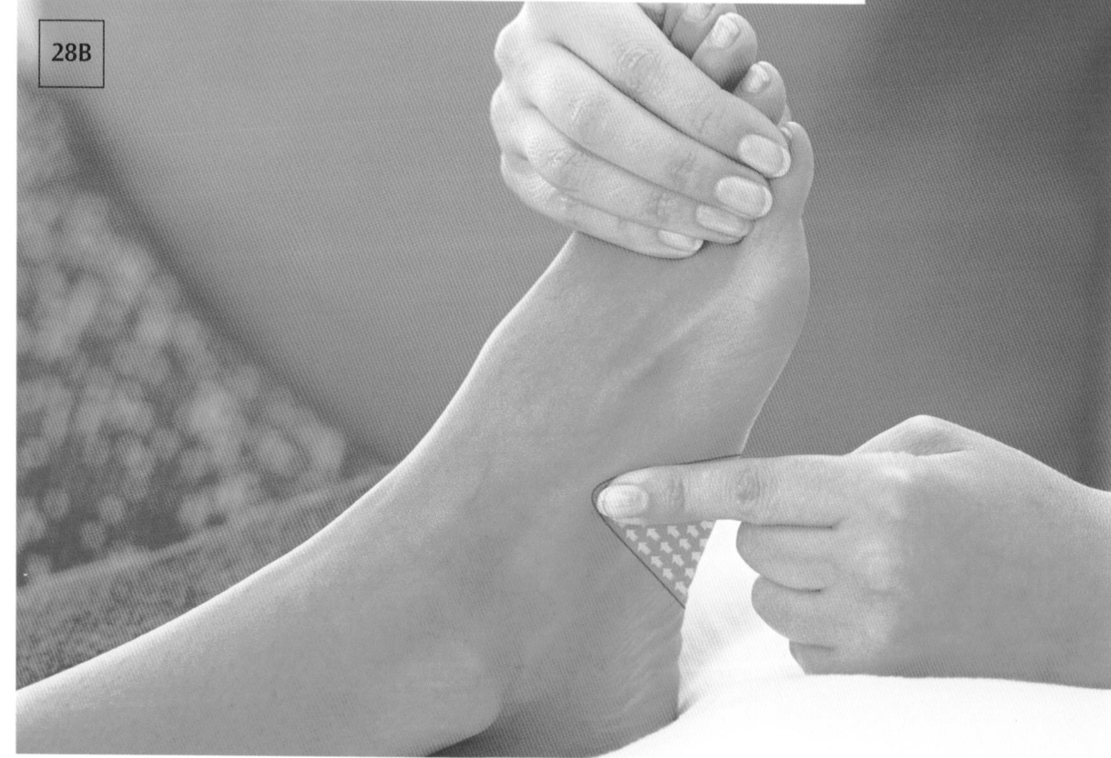

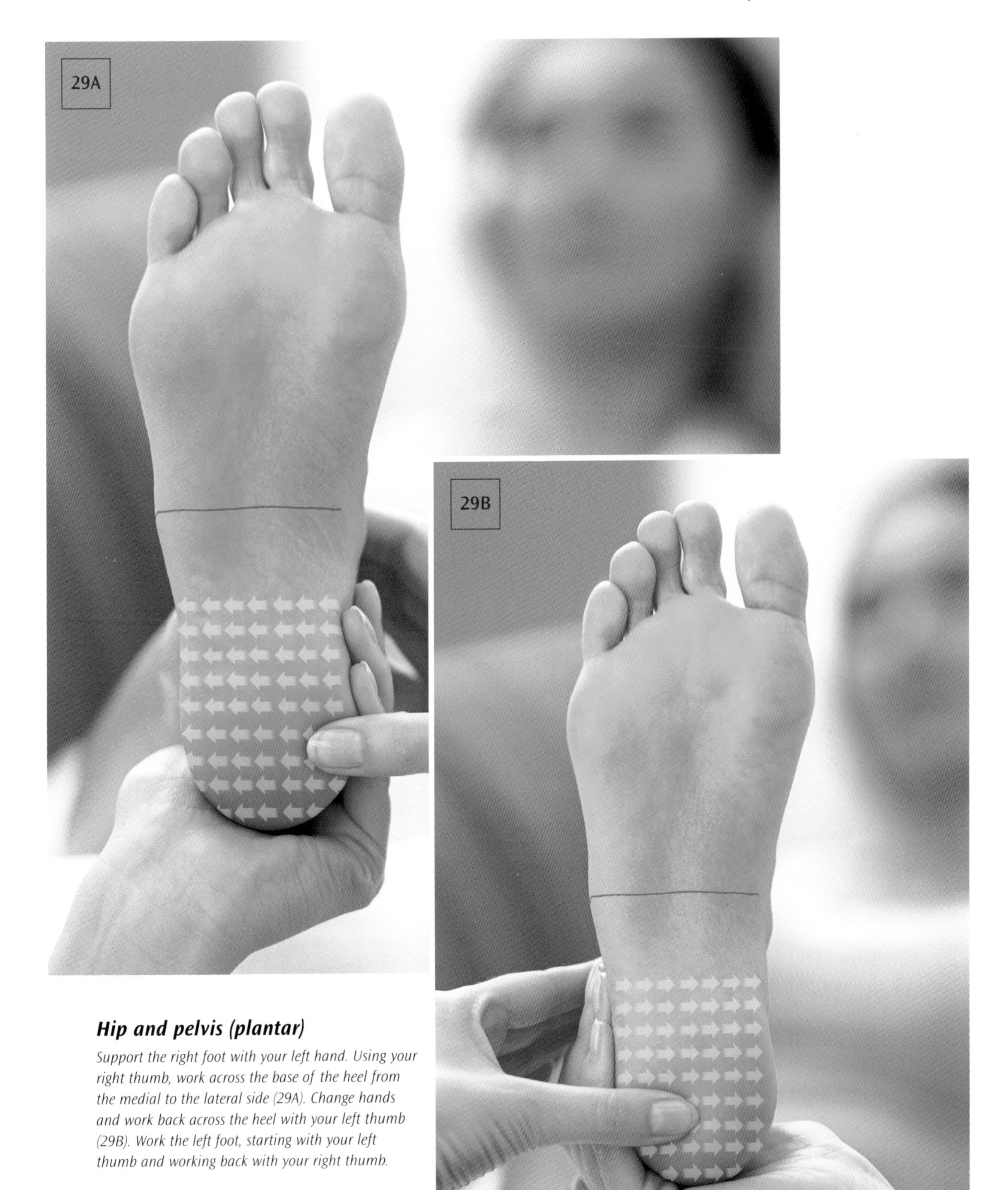

Hip and pelvis (plantar)

Support the right foot with your left hand. Using your right thumb, work across the base of the heel from the medial to the lateral side (29A). Change hands and work back across the heel with your left thumb (29B). Work the left foot, starting with your left thumb and working back with your right thumb.

Primary sciatic

Support the top of the right foot with your right hand. Using your left index finger, work the area behind the ankle bone (30A). Continue creeping about 1½ inches (4 cm) up the ankle (30B). Switch hands to work the left foot.

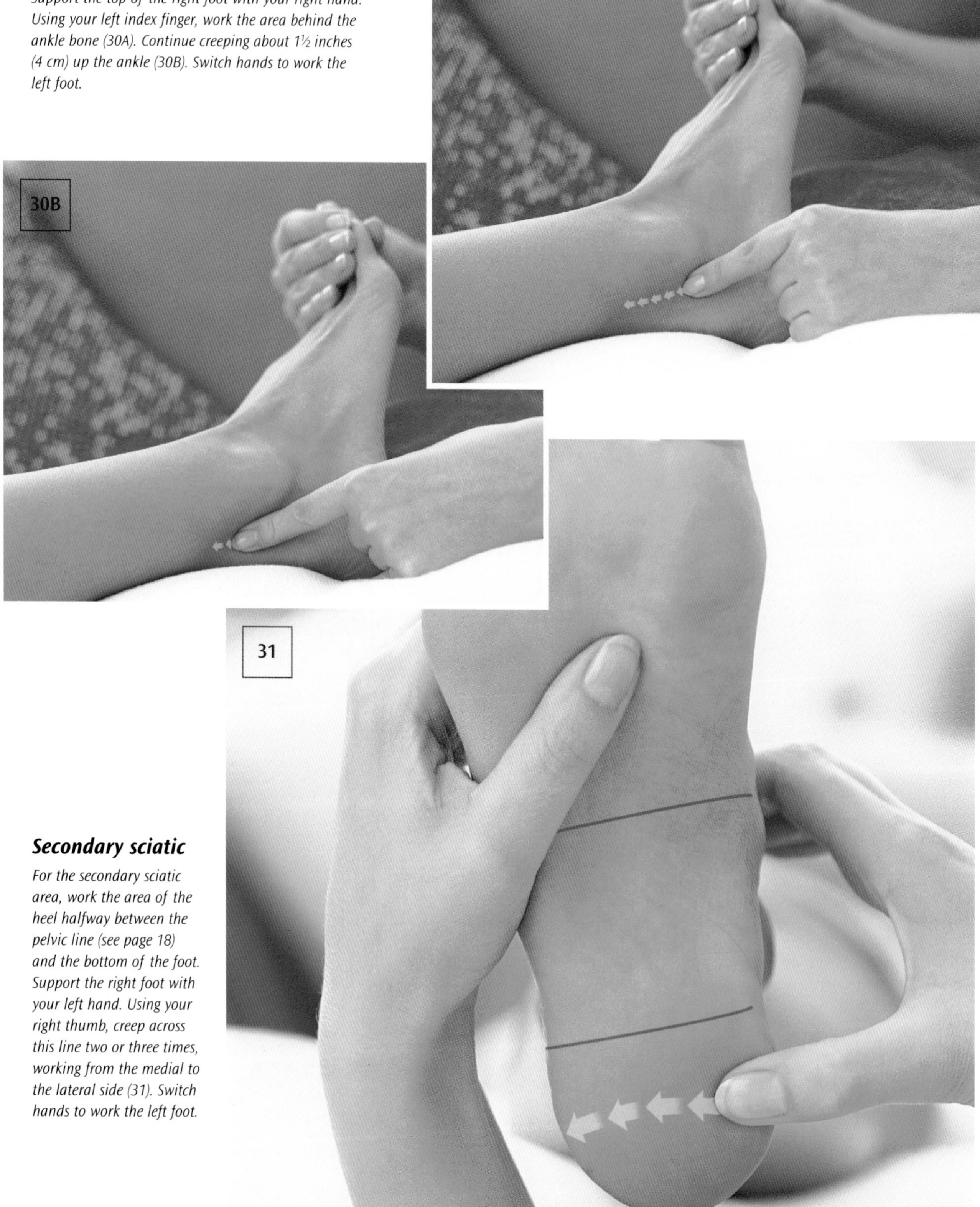

Secondary sciatic

For the secondary sciatic area, work the area of the heel halfway between the pelvic line (see page 18) and the bottom of the foot. Support the right foot with your left hand. Using your right thumb, creep across this line two or three times, working from the medial to the lateral side (31). Switch hands to work the left foot.

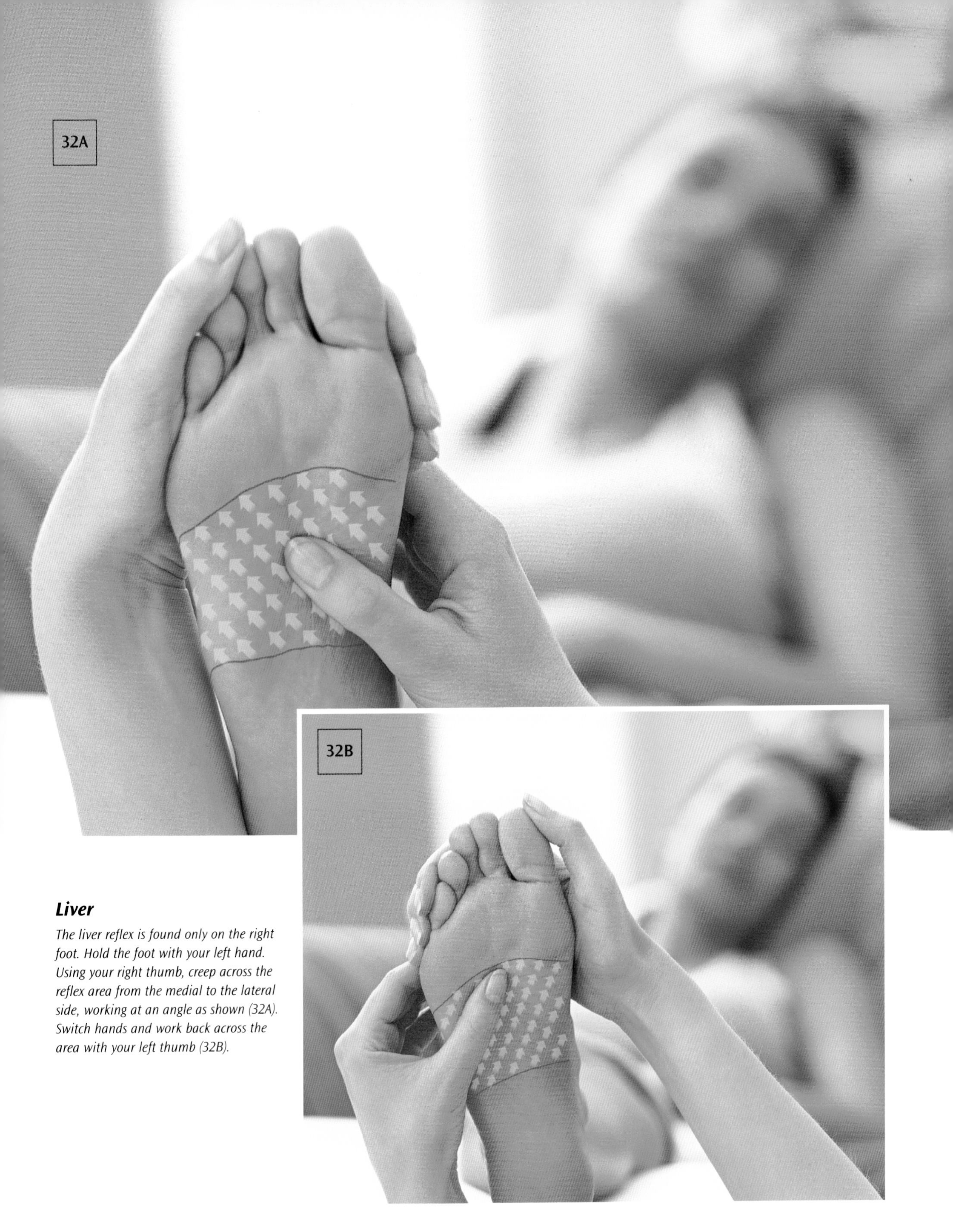

Liver

The liver reflex is found only on the right foot. Hold the foot with your left hand. Using your right thumb, creep across the reflex area from the medial to the lateral side, working at an angle as shown (32A). Switch hands and work back across the area with your left thumb (32B).

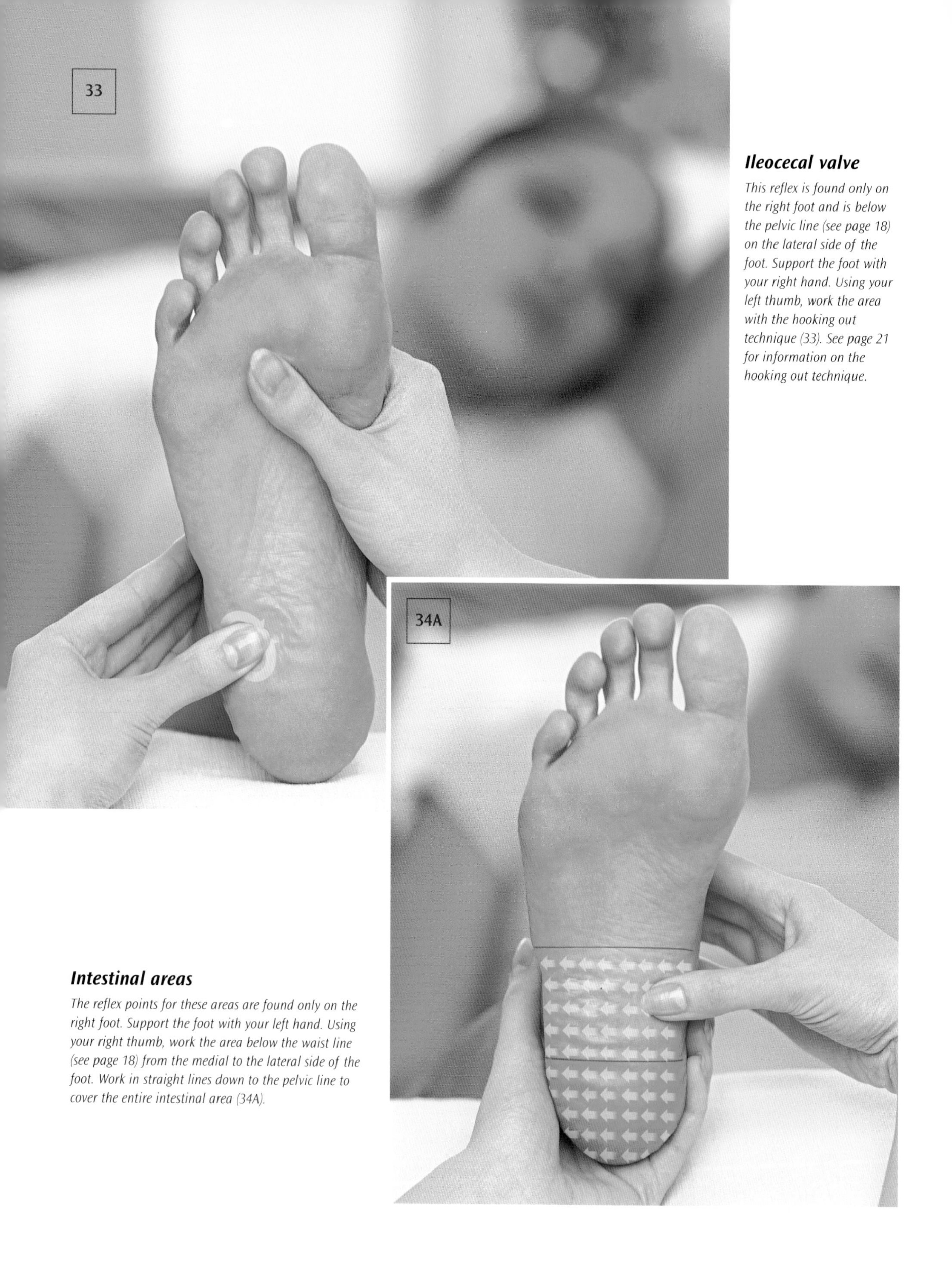

Ileocecal valve

This reflex is found only on the right foot and is below the pelvic line (see page 18) on the lateral side of the foot. Support the foot with your right hand. Using your left thumb, work the area with the hooking out technique (33). See page 21 for information on the hooking out technique.

Intestinal areas

The reflex points for these areas are found only on the right foot. Support the foot with your left hand. Using your right thumb, work the area below the waist line (see page 18) from the medial to the lateral side of the foot. Work in straight lines down to the pelvic line to cover the entire intestinal area (34A).

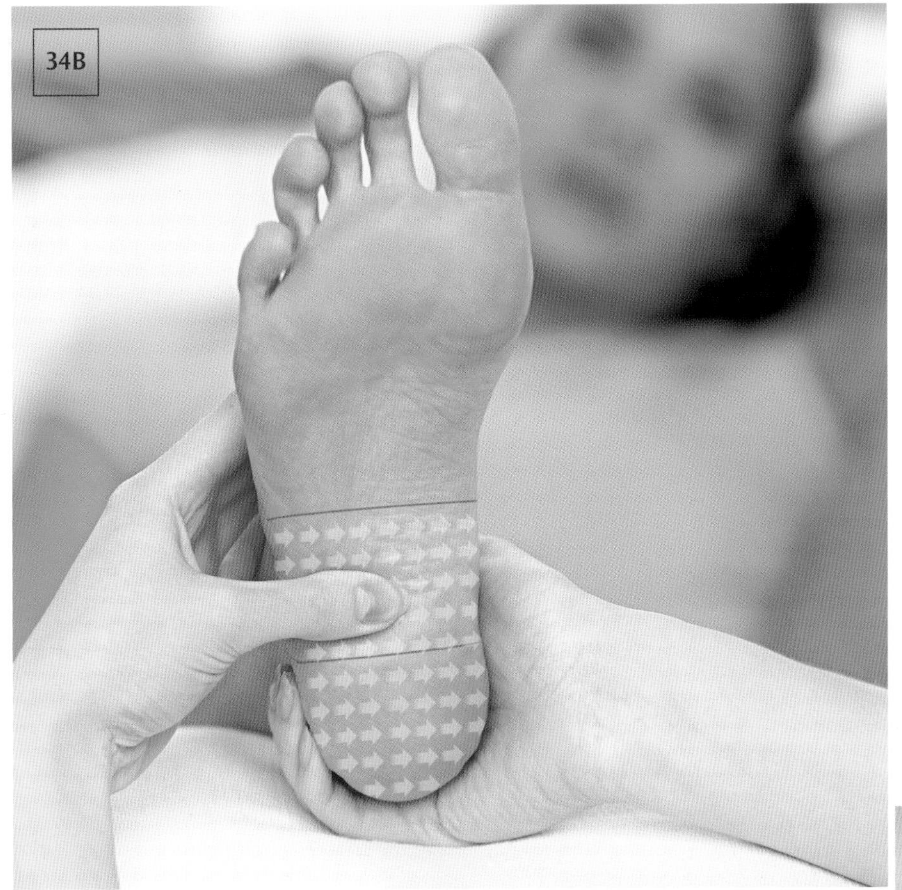

Intestinal areas

Support the foot in your right hand. Using your left thumb, work back across the area below the waist line, this time from the lateral to the medial side of the foot (34B). Work in straight lines down to the pelvic line as before.

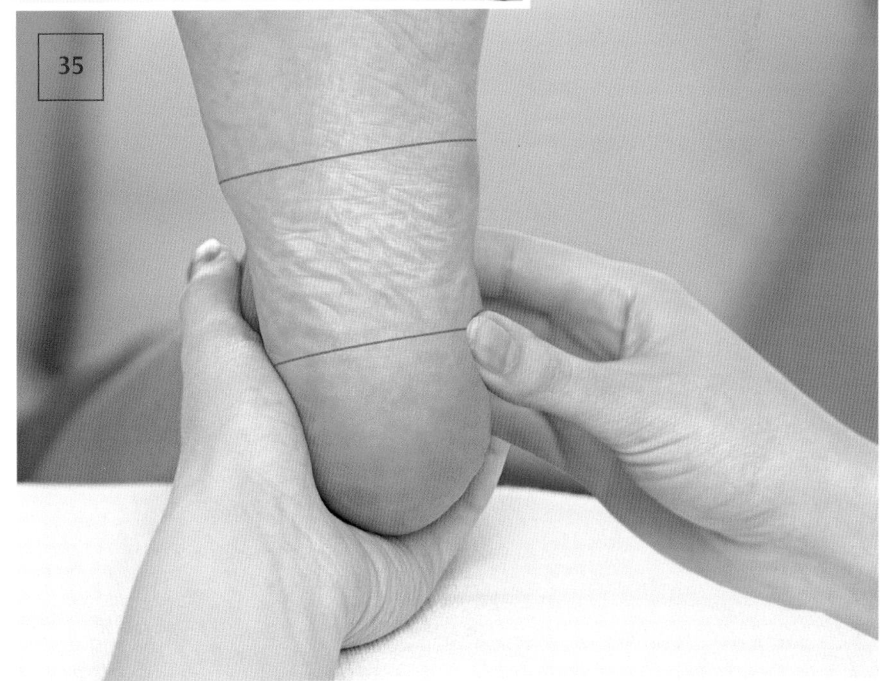

Bladder

Support the right foot with your left hand. Using your right thumb, isolate the soft puffy area on the medial side of the foot (35) and work over this area two or three times. Switch hands to work the left foot.

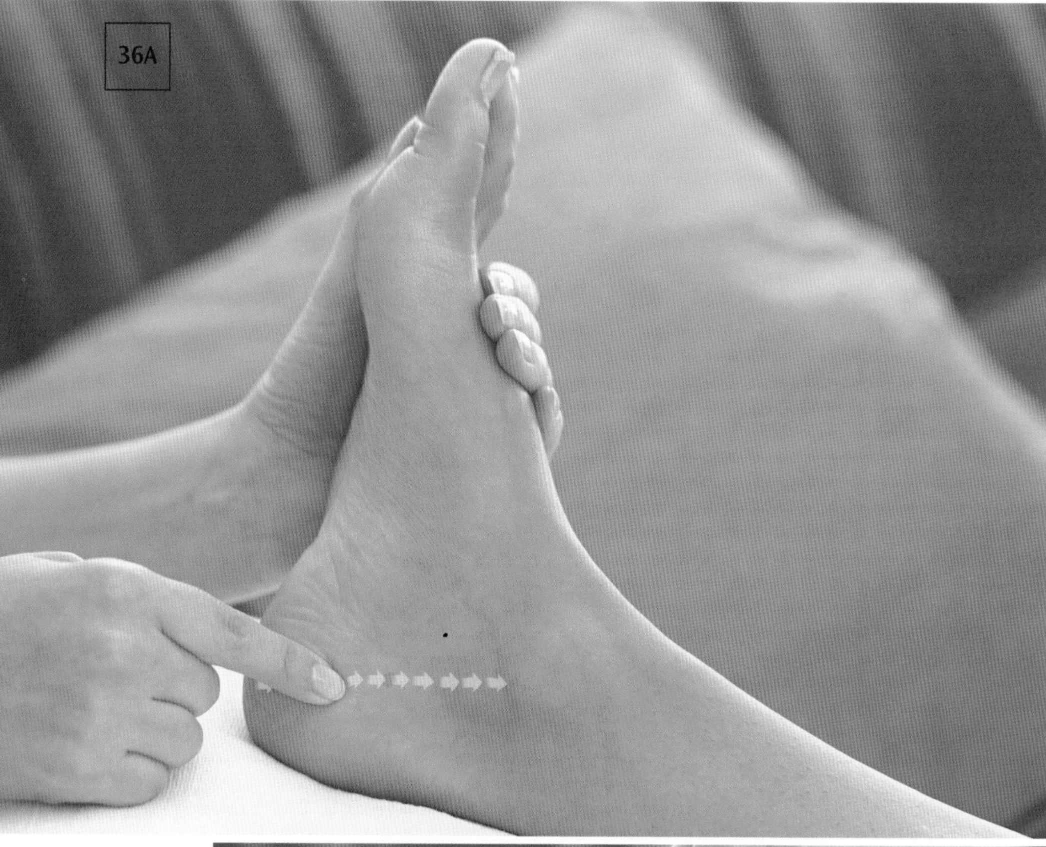

Uterus/Prostate

The reflex point for the uterus/prostate is between the heel and the ankle bone on the medial side of the foot. Support the right foot with your left hand. Using your right index finger, work from the tip of the heel to the ankle bone (36A, 36B). Switch hands to work the left foot.

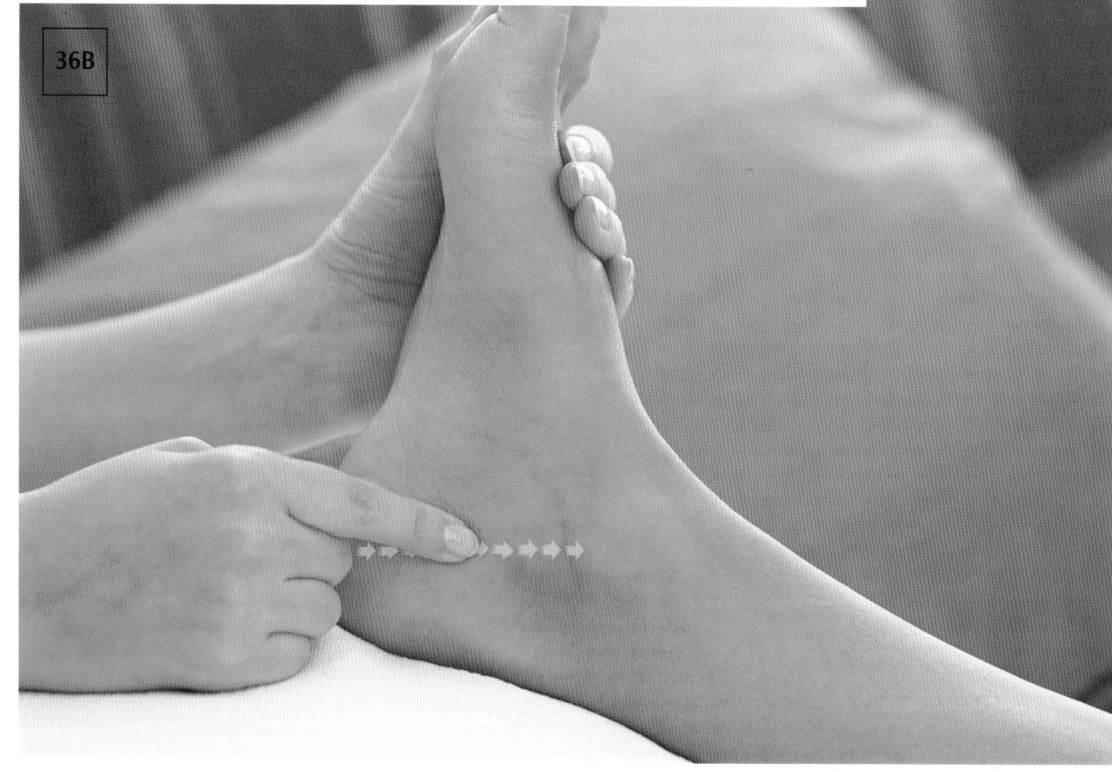

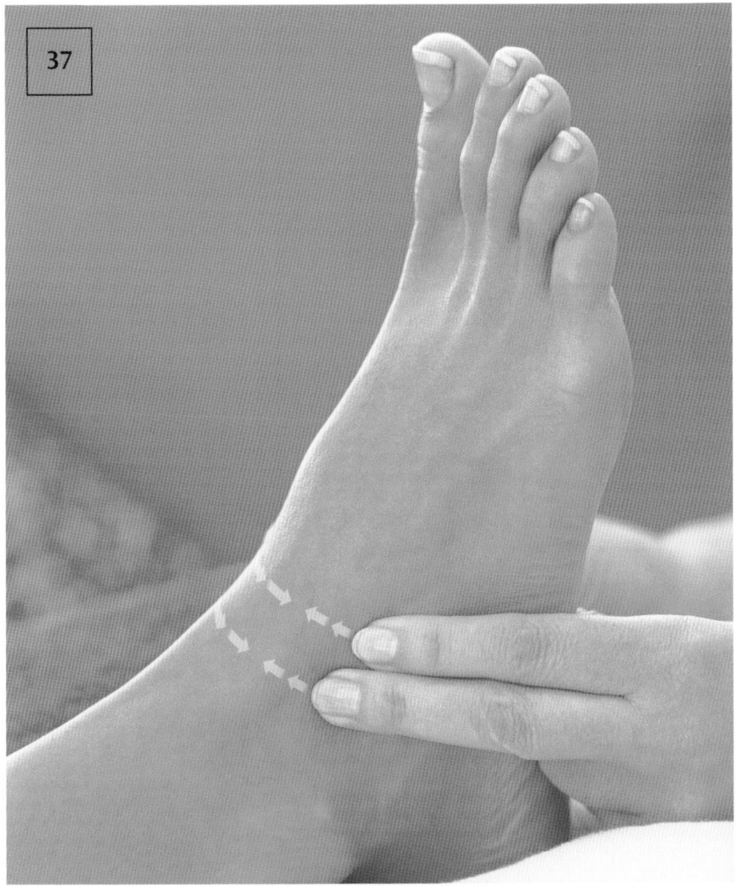

Fallopian tubes/Vas deferens

Press into the sole of the right foot with both thumbs. At the same time, creep across the top of the foot with the index and third fingers of both hands (37). Repeat two or three times. Switch hands to work the left foot.

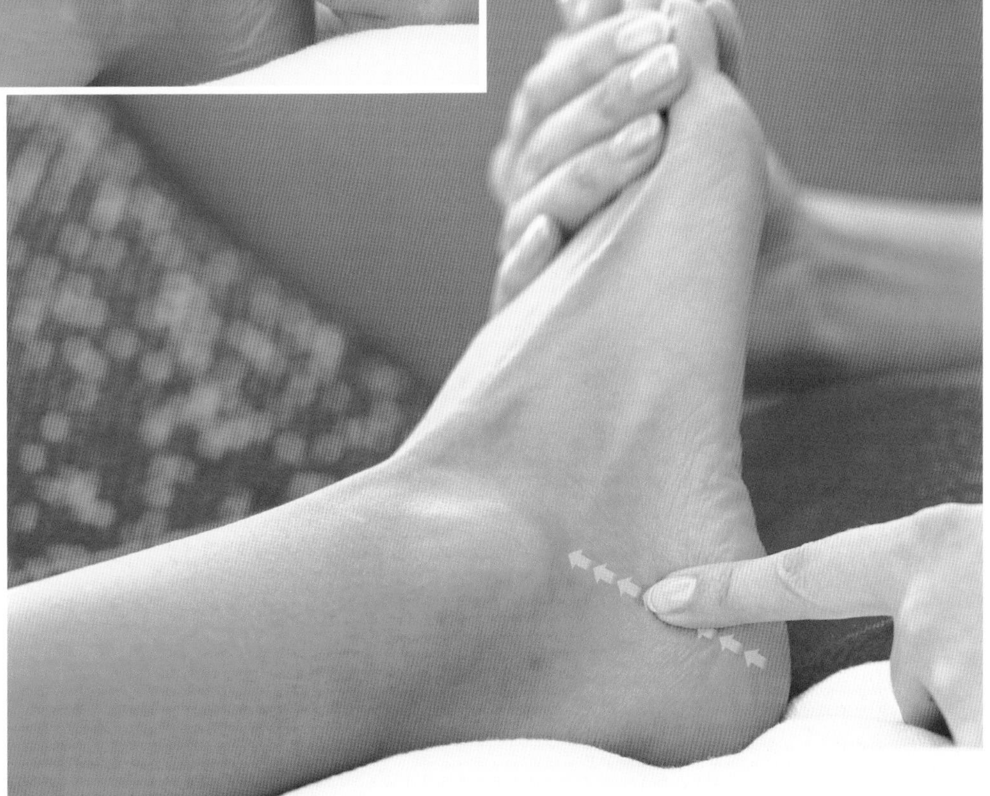

Ovary/Testis

The reflex point for the ovary/testis is between the tip of the heel and the ankle bone on the lateral side of the foot. Support the right foot in your right hand. Using your left index finger, creep from the tip of the heel to the ankle bone (38). Switch hands to work the left foot.

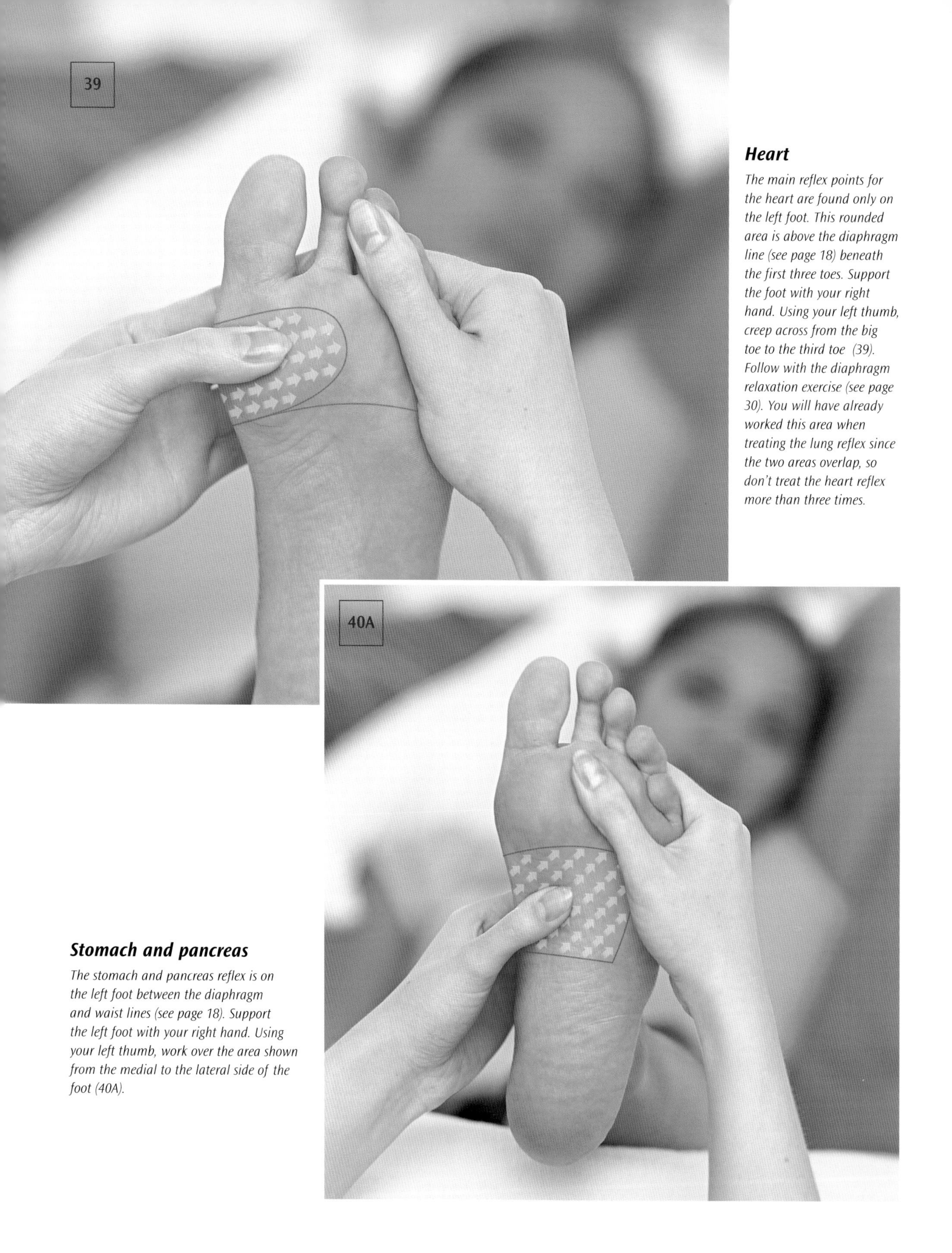

Heart

The main reflex points for the heart are found only on the left foot. This rounded area is above the diaphragm line (see page 18) beneath the first three toes. Support the foot with your right hand. Using your left thumb, creep across from the big toe to the third toe (39). Follow with the diaphragm relaxation exercise (see page 30). You will have already worked this area when treating the lung reflex since the two areas overlap, so don't treat the heart reflex more than three times.

Stomach and pancreas

The stomach and pancreas reflex is on the left foot between the diaphragm and waist lines (see page 18). Support the left foot with your right hand. Using your left thumb, work over the area shown from the medial to the lateral side of the foot (40A).

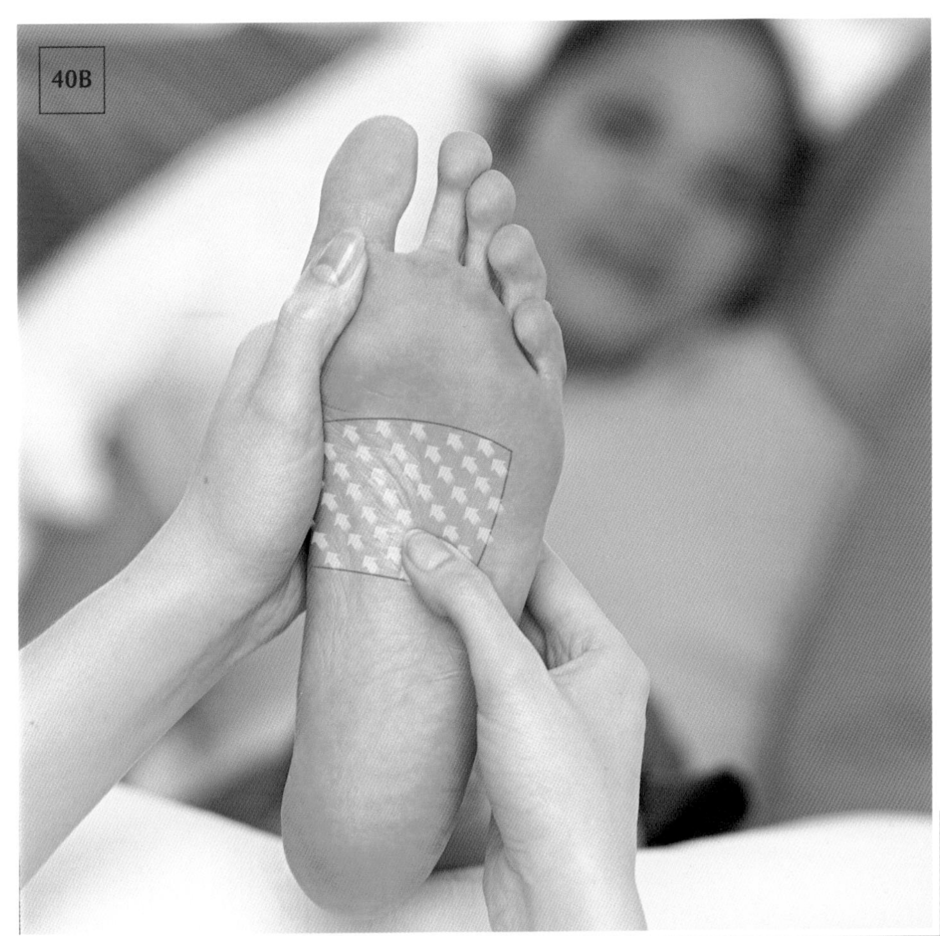

Stomach and pancreas

Swap hands and work back from the lateral to the medial side with your right thumb (40B).

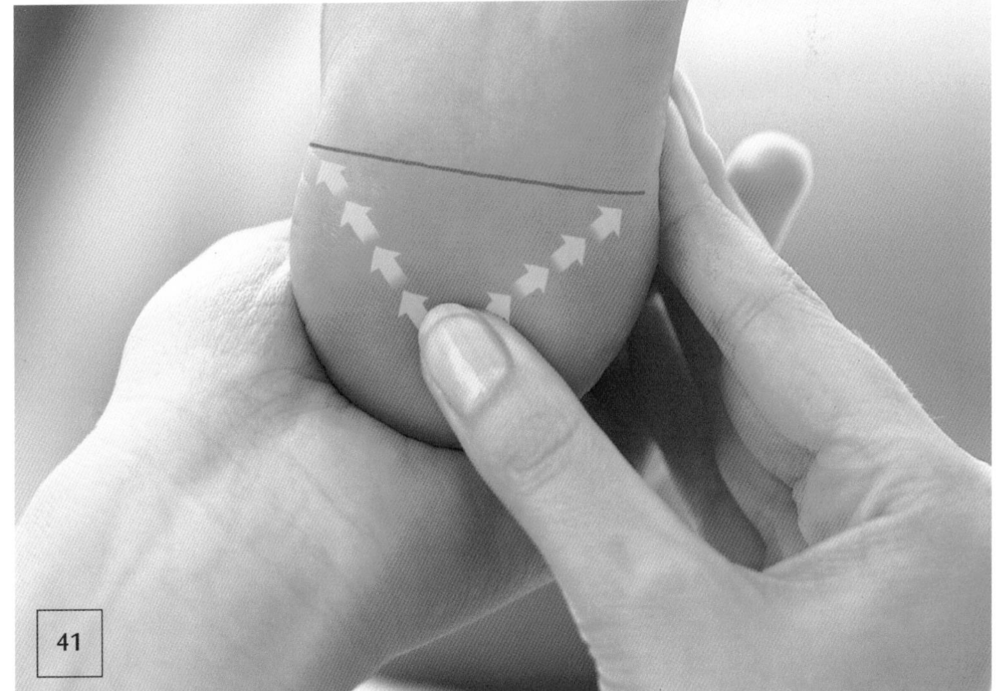

Sigmoid colon and rectum

This is a V-shaped reflex area under the pelvic line (see page 18) and is found only on the left foot. Support the foot with your right hand. Use the thumb of your left hand to work up the outside fork of the reflex area. Switch hands and use your right thumb to work up the inside fork (41).

Winding down

A relaxing massage after reflexology relaxes the receiver and can increase the benefits of the treatment. Ask the receiver to lie down on a firm, flat surface. Use a little oil on your hands.

■ Using your index fingers, work up the spine again, making small, circular movements (5). Do this twice. Finish by sliding your palms from the base of the spine to the shoulders (6).

■ Using the palms of your hands, massage the shoulders with gentle, circular movements (1). Work across to either side of the spine (2). Massage the neck with the tips of your index fingers (3).

■ Again using the palms of your hands, massage either side of the spine with gentle, circular movements. Start at the base of the spine and work up (4).

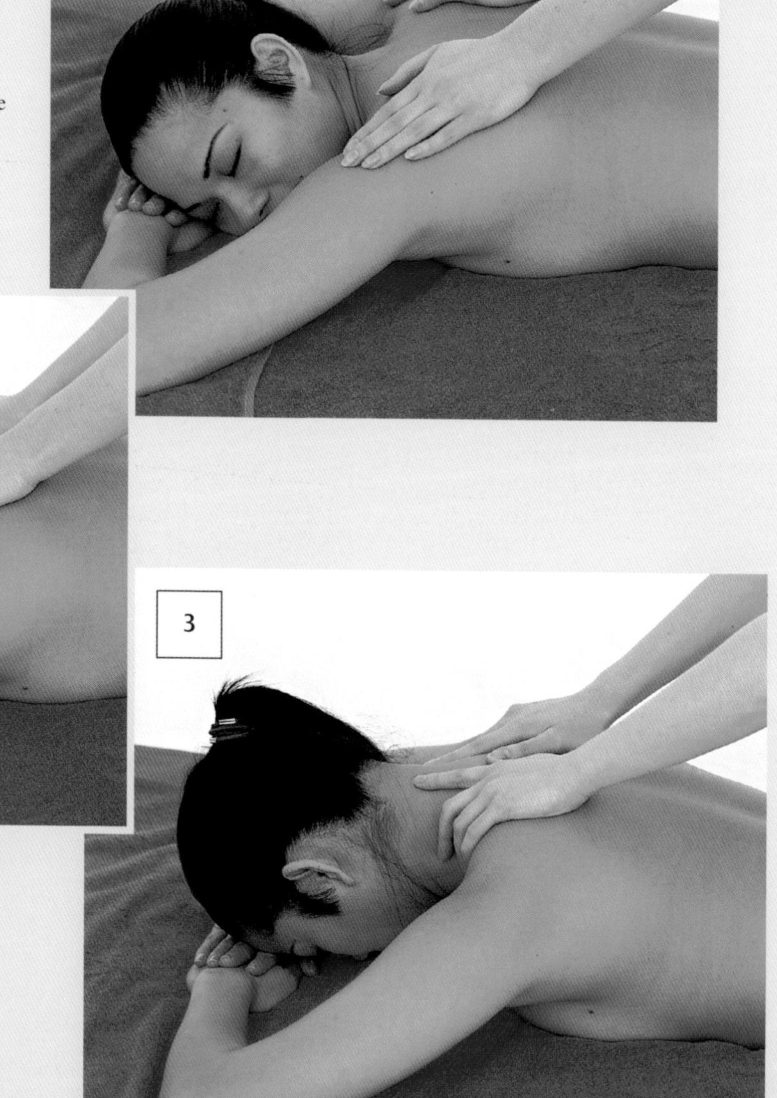

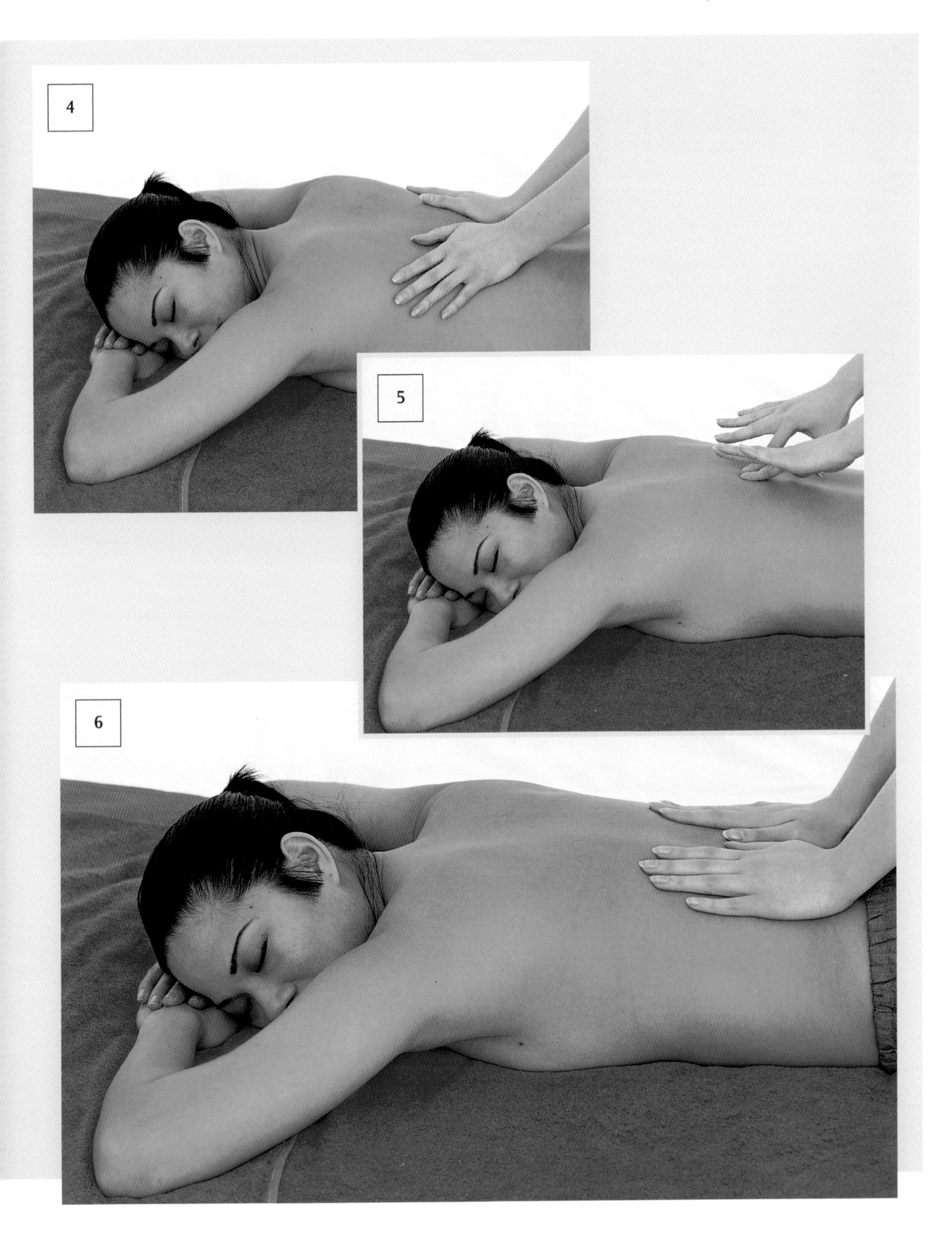
4
5
6

TREATING NECK PAIN

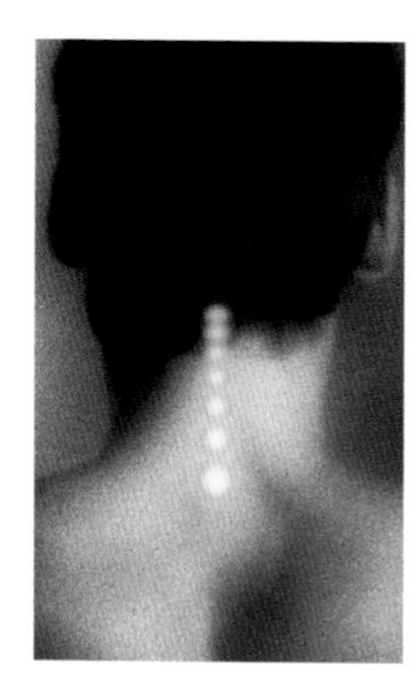

Cervical spine
The cervical spine starts at the base of the skull. These seven vertebrae support the skull and allow a wide range of head movements.

The seven vertebrae in the neck are called the cervical vertebrae. They support the weight of the head and allow the neck to be very flexible. The top two cervical vertebrae are known as the atlas and the axis and they enable the head to nod and turn. Just think how many times in a day you move your head like this.

Neck pain is not as common as lower back pain. However, the neck is less well protected than the rest of the spine, so it is vulnerable to problems from injury, wear and tear, and degenerative diseases.

Treating pain, stiffness, and tension in the neck by foot reflexology is a wonderful way to relieve discomfort. Reflexology can free muscular tension, improve circulation, and restore the normal functioning of the neck.

Causes of neck pain

Pain, stiffness, and discomfort in your neck may be caused by accidents, such as whiplash after a car crash, falls, or simply by general tension. Sitting at a computer screen for long periods, for example, can make the muscles, ligaments, and joints on either side of your neck feel tense and irritated.

Degenerative diseases such as osteoarthritis and rheumatoid arthritis (see page 12) can cause wear and damage in the neck, resulting in pain. Put your hand at the back of your neck and you'll feel the seventh cervical vertebra, where your neck joins your shoulders. This is the most prominent of the cervical vertebrae, and it endures a lot of wear, and consequently often becomes arthritic with age.

Cervical disc degeneration is another cause of neck pain. As you get older, the discs between the bones in the neck can come under stress and become damaged. This can result in a herniated cervical disc—the core of a disc starts to protrude, putting pressure on the spinal cord or nerves (see page 94).

Neck tension

If you stop what you're doing for a moment and think about your neck, you'll probably find you're holding it very rigidly. Everyone holds tension in the neck and when you're stressed, it can feel like you're carrying the weight of the world on your shoulders. Sitting hunched over a desk, holding the

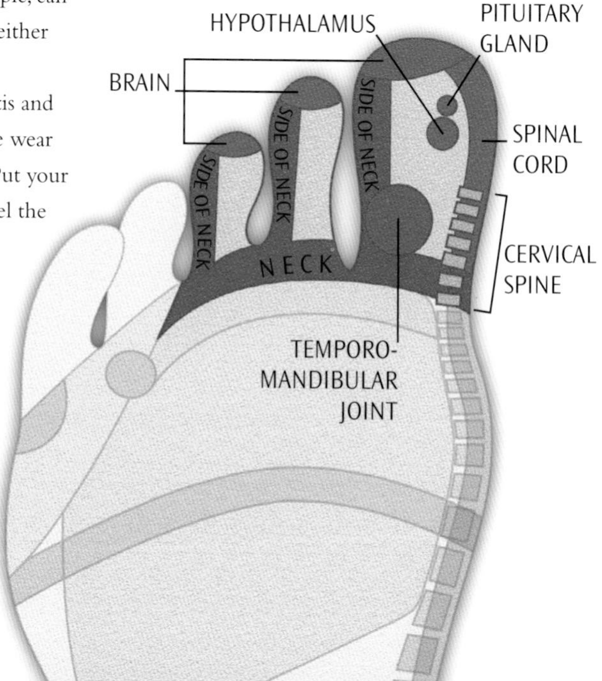

Areas on the foot
The reflex areas for the neck are on the big toe and second and third toes, so work on these areas to treat neck problems.

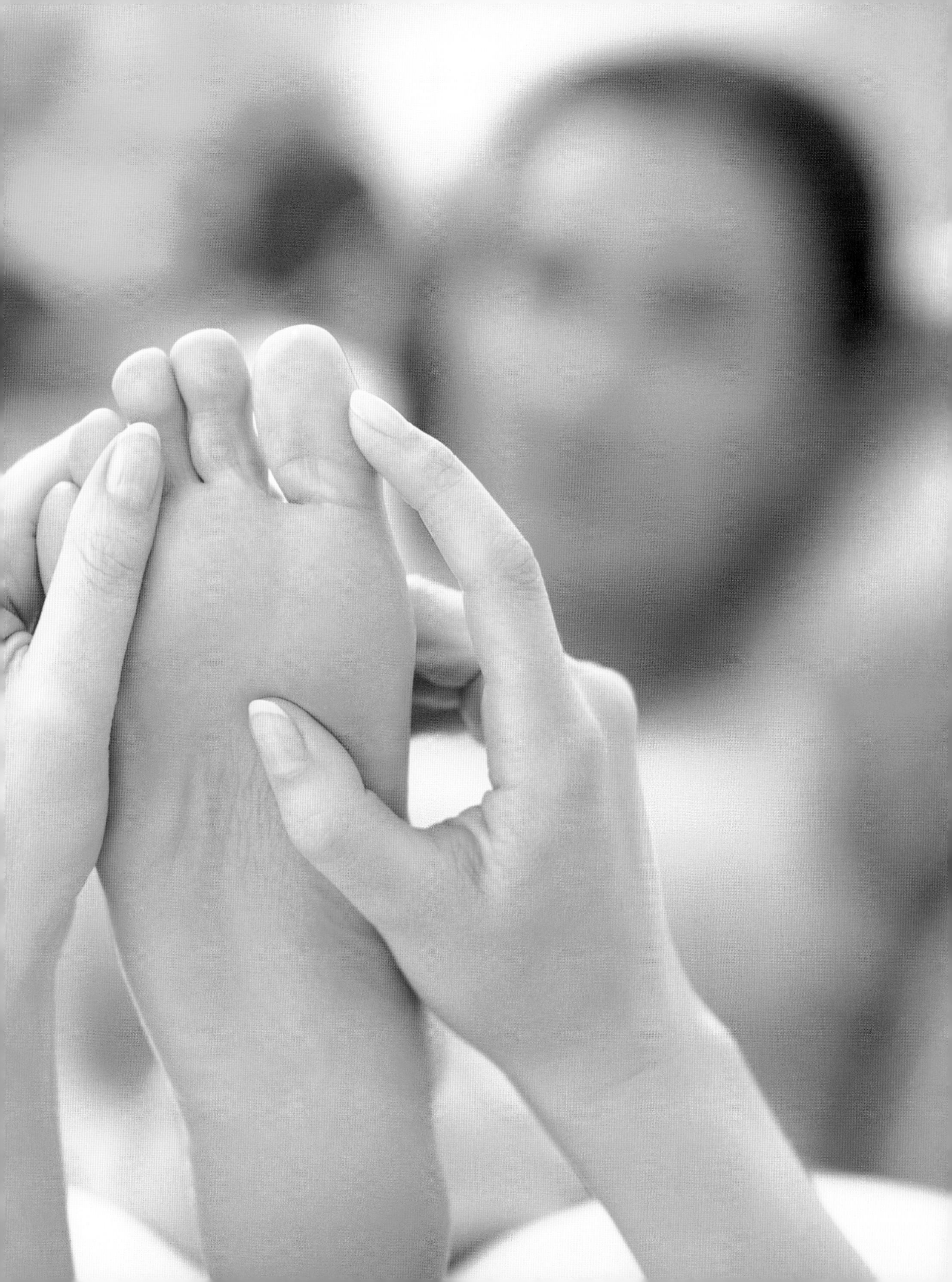

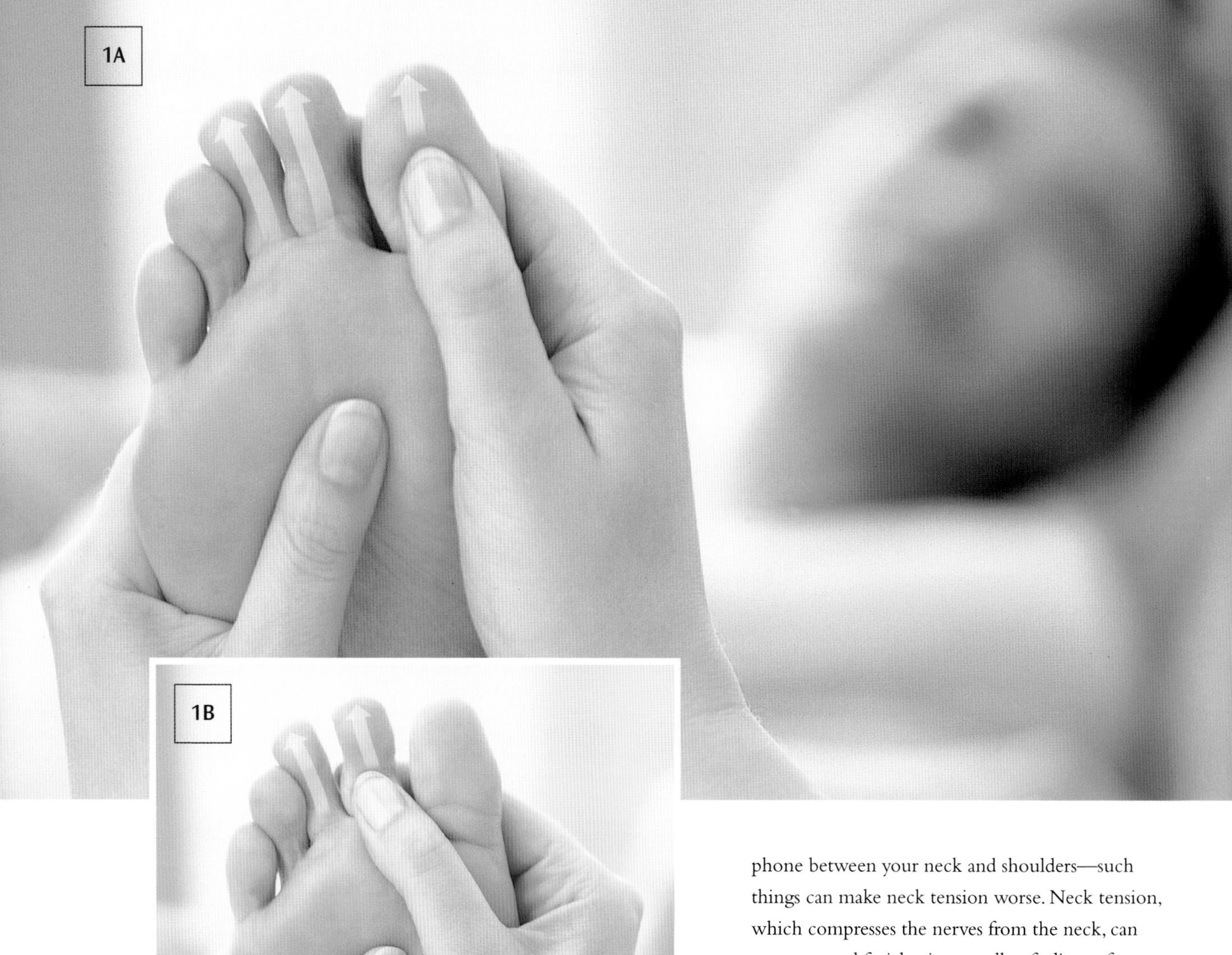

Neck and head

To treat all areas from the back of the neck to the top of the head, apply pressure to the underside of the big toe (1A) and to the second and third toes (1B, 1C). The third toe represents the side of the head in line with the ear.

phone between your neck and shoulders—such things can make neck tension worse. Neck tension, which compresses the nerves from the neck, can cause ear and facial pain, as well as feelings of dizziness and confusion. There are theories that it could even be a cause of dementia in later life.

Reducing neck tension

To reduce tension, keep your neck moving. Rotating your head—looking from right to left, up to the ceiling and down to the ground—will help to ease general stiffness.

At night, use a postural support orthopedic pillow to keep your head in a good position as you sleep. Sleeping on a pillow that's too high can put extra strain on the muscles and ligaments in your neck and increase neck tension.

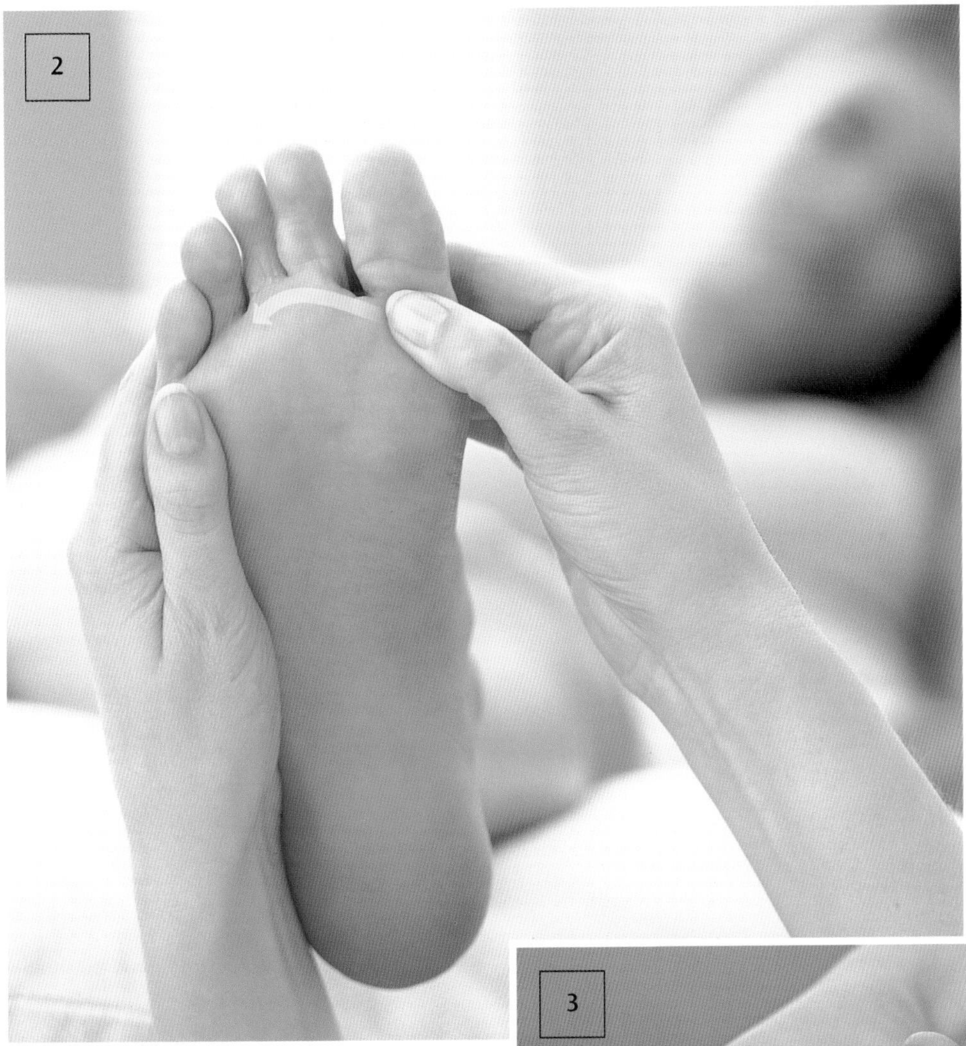

Back of the neck

To treat the base of the neck, (the area that joins the head to the shoulders), support the right foot with your left hand. Using your right thumb, creep along the base of the first three toes (the shoulder line) three times (2). Switch hands to treat the left foot.

Front of the neck

To treat the front of the neck, make a fist with your left hand and place it against the upper part of the right foot. With your right index finger, creep along the bases of the first three toes (3). Switch hands to treat the left foot.

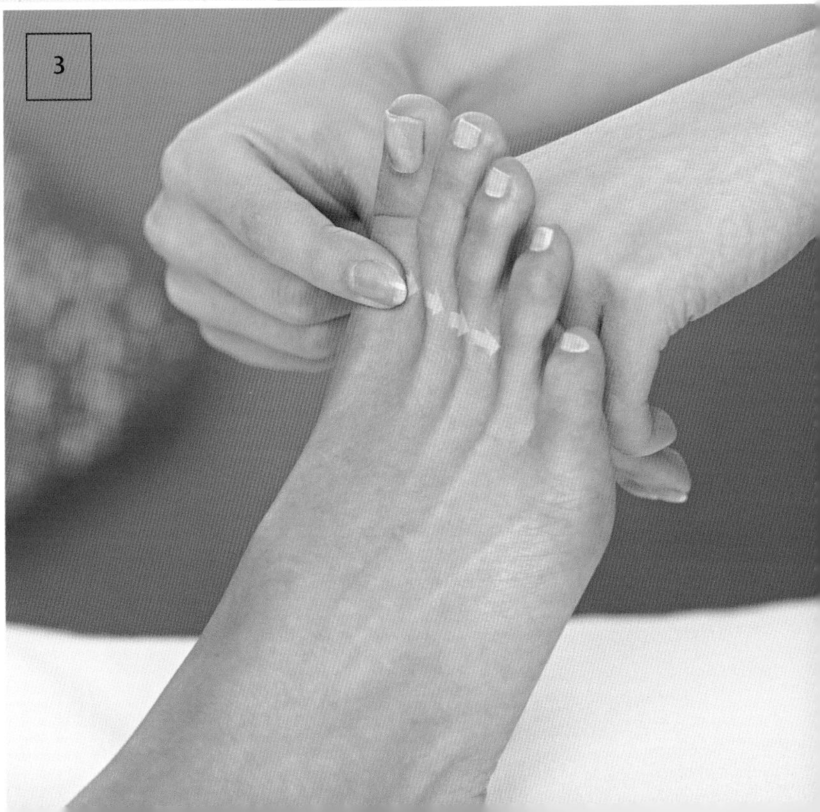

Wry neck

At some time, nearly everyone has woken up in the morning with a stiff neck and the feeling that it's difficult to turn the head to the right or left. This condition is called wry neck and affects the facet joints—the places where vertebrae link together. Wry neck may be caused by strenuous activity the day before, such as a grueling game of tennis or squash. Swimming breaststroke can also be a cause. Breaststroke can strain the neck, because many people swim with the head in an upright position, and it's not recommended for anyone suffering from neck problems.

Wry neck may also come following a restless night when you toss and turn in your bed after a

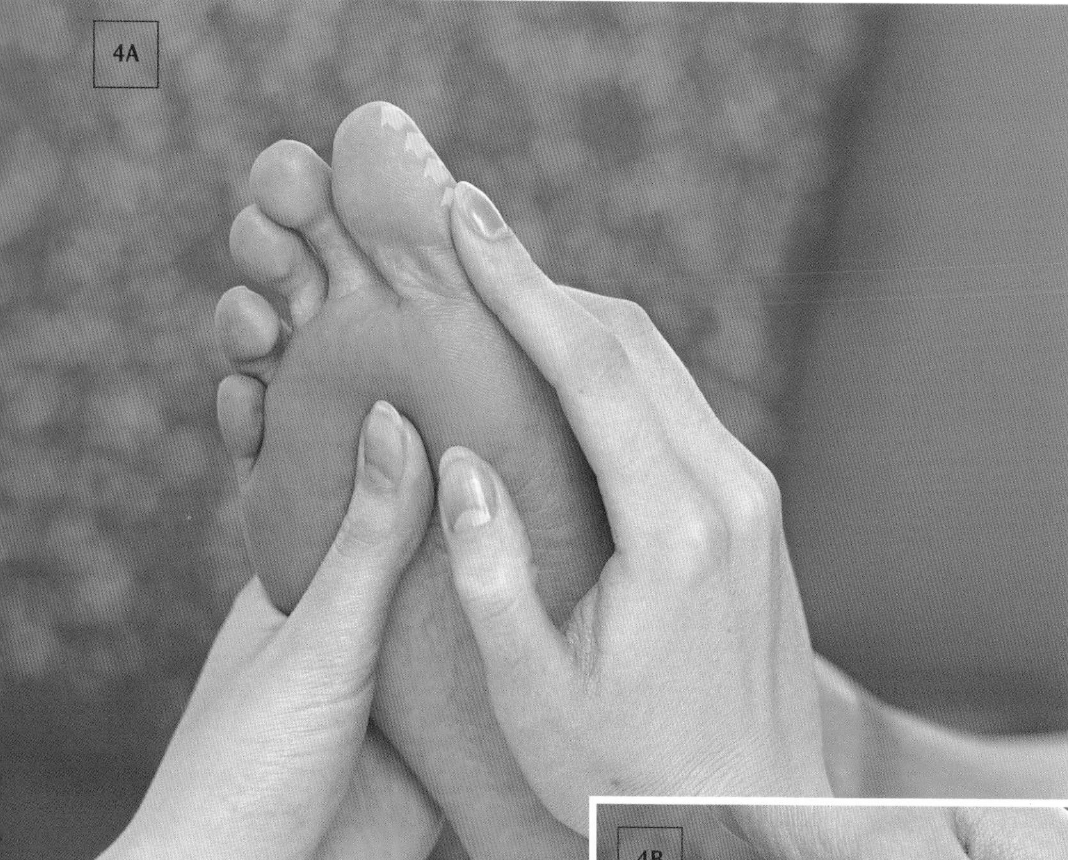

Neck conditions

Working the prominent parts of the seven cervical vertebrae is helpful for relieving conditions such as arthritis in the neck or damage from whiplash injury following a car accident.

Support the right foot with your left hand. Using your right index finger, creep up the medial side of the foot (4A). Switch hands to treat the left foot.

Supporting the right foot with the back of your right hand, work down the outer edge of the big toe with your left thumb (4B). Switch hands to treat the left foot.

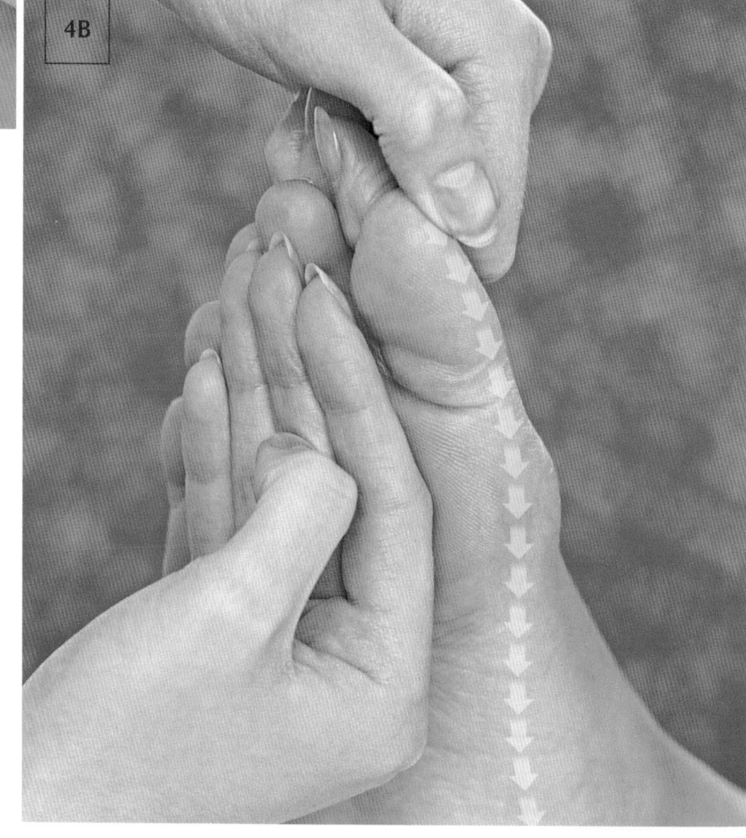

bad dream or worrying over emotional and stressful situations from the previous day.

Neuralgia

Neuralgia is a severe shooting, burning, or stabbing pain, often following the course of a nerve in the head or neck. This type of pain may start after you've had a tooth taken out or if you've been unlucky enough to have shingles affecting the face, although there's not always an obvious cause. Pains may come and go without warning, and last for minutes or hours. Treatment by reflexology can bring great relief from this unpleasant and painful condition.

If the neuralgia is caused by shingles, dabbing the area with a cotton ball soaked in lavender oil can be very soothing.

Neck conditions

Use your thumb to work down the lateral side of the big toe (5A), and then the second and third toes (5B, 5C). Use your right thumb on the right foot, and your left thumb on the left foot as before. This helps to relieve neck pain from arthritis as well as from whiplash injury.

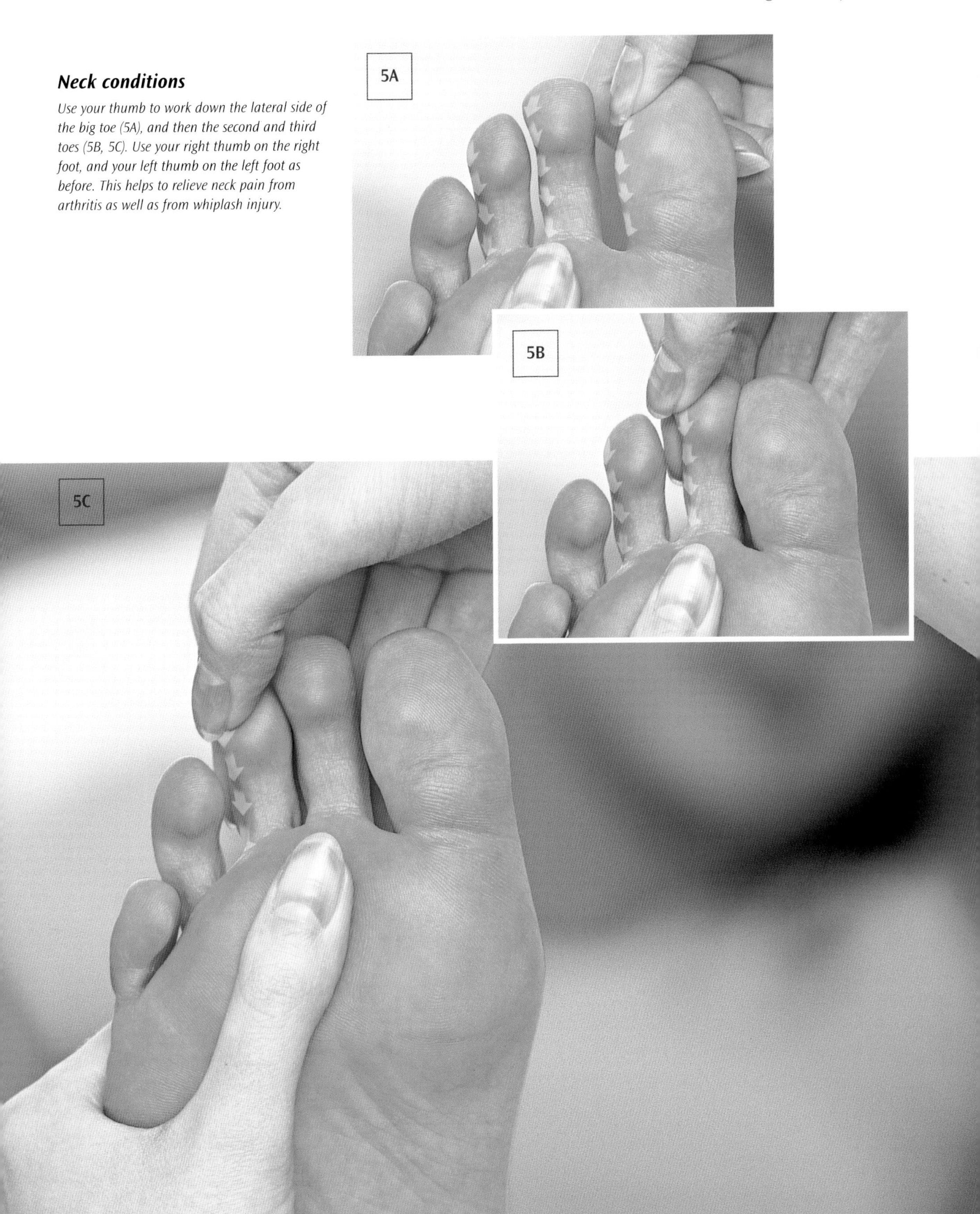

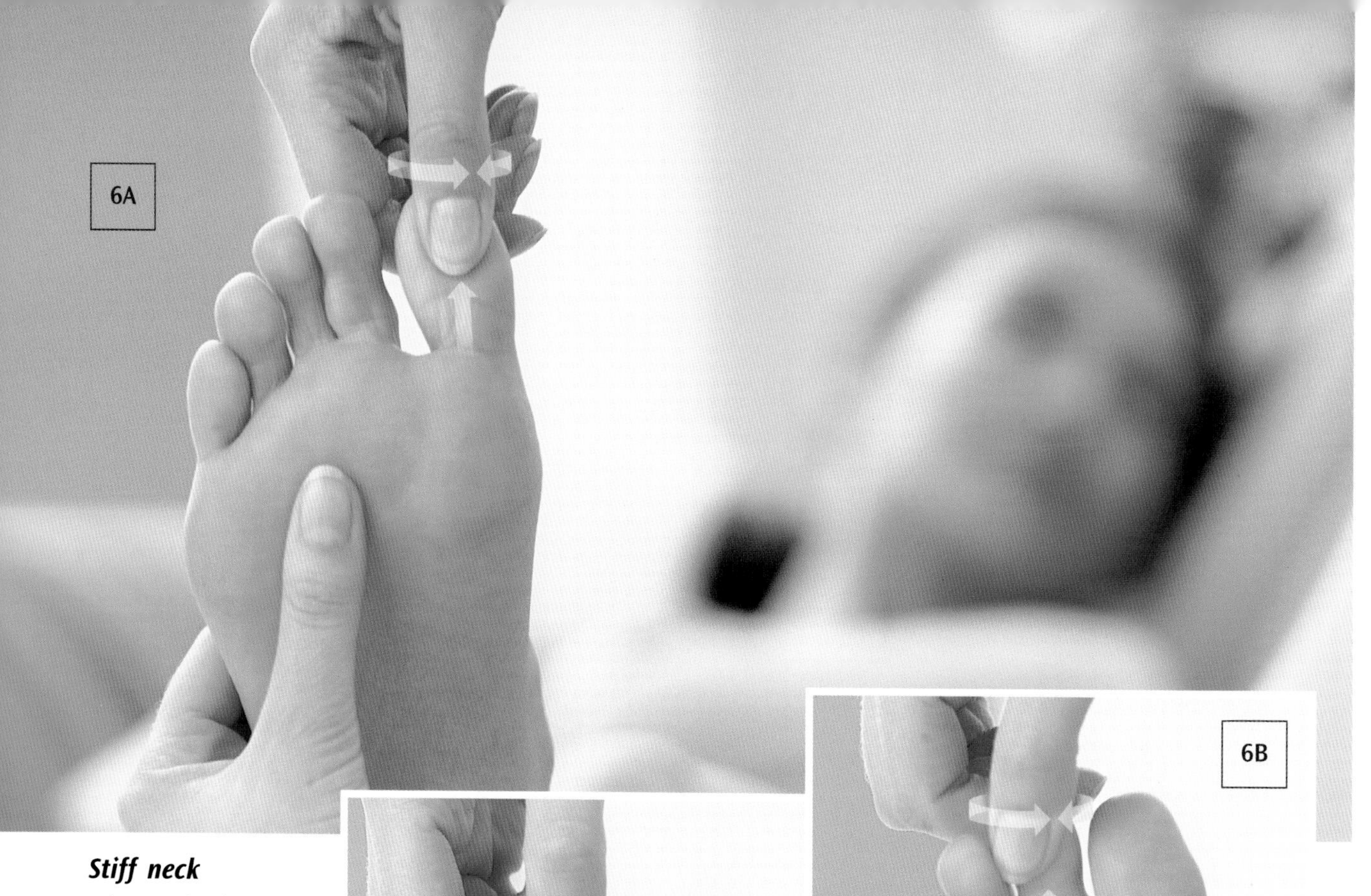

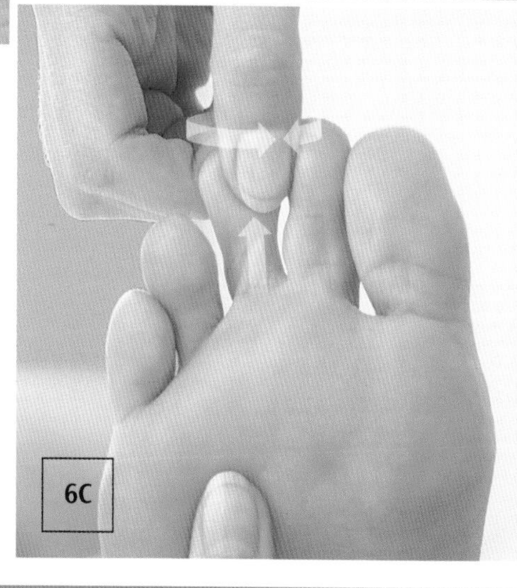

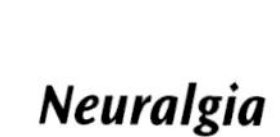

Stiff neck

Using your thumb, gently support and lift each of the first three toes and rotate in an inward direction (6A, 6B, 6C). Use your right thumb on the right foot, and your left thumb on the left foot.

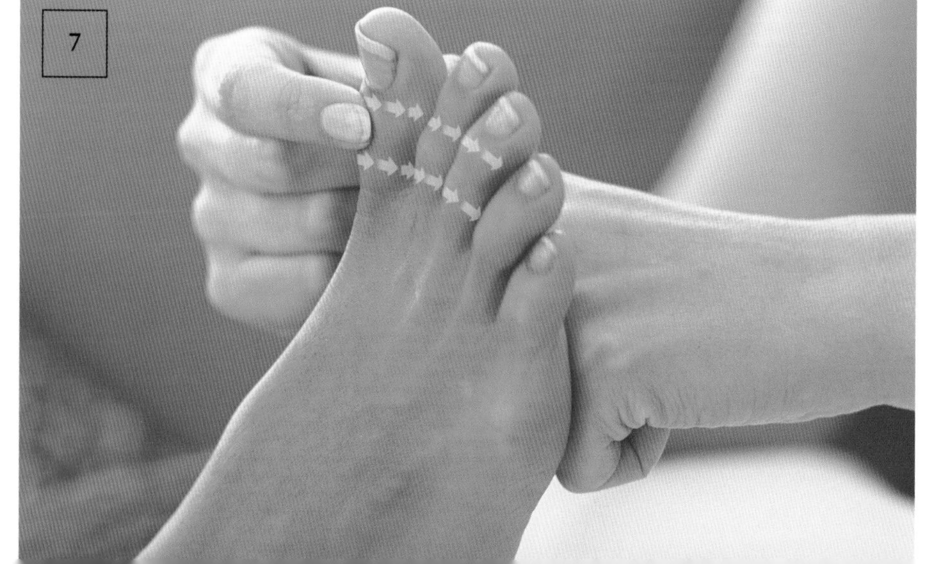

Neuralgia

To relieve face pain, make a fist with your left hand and place it against the upper part of the right foot. With your right index finger, creep along the front of the first three toes. When treating the left foot, rest the foot against your right fist and use your left index finger to creep along the toes (7).

Simple neck exercises

Take care of your neck. If you have to sit or stand for long periods during the day, stop from time to time and gently turn your neck from side to side to release tension and keep your neck strong and flexible (1, 2).

Even if you're suffering from pain and stiffness in your neck, always try to keep moving. Gently rotate your head, looking up at the ceiling and down at the floor to keep muscles and ligaments supple (3, 4). If you don't move, your neck will stiffen further, weakening the ligaments and muscles, and causing yet more problems.

Another good way of relieving neck pain is this gentle form of self traction. Lie on your back on your bed with your head hanging over the foot of the bed (5). Remain lying in this position for at least five minutes to stretch out the tension in your neck muscles.

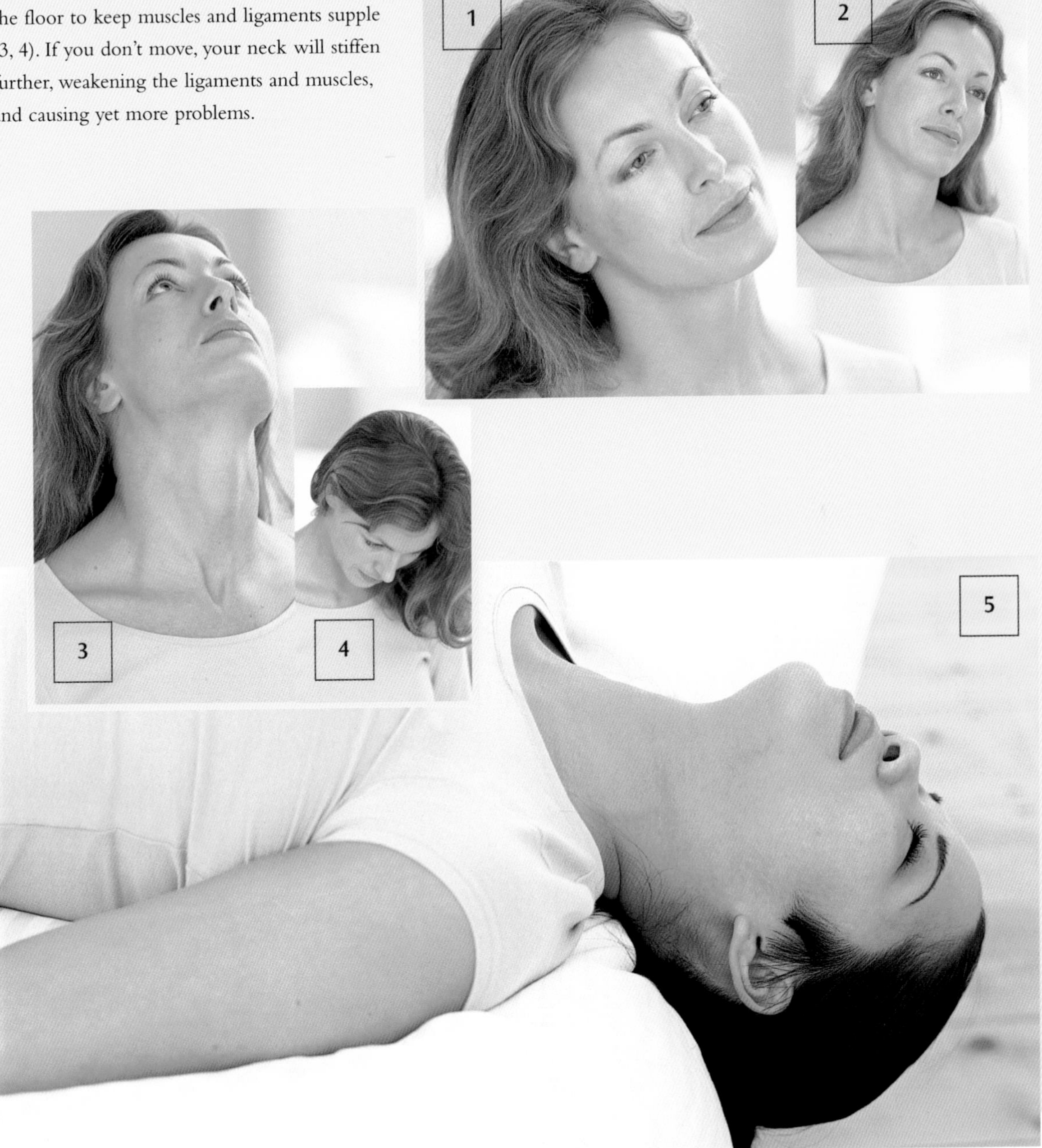

TREATING THE UPPER BACK

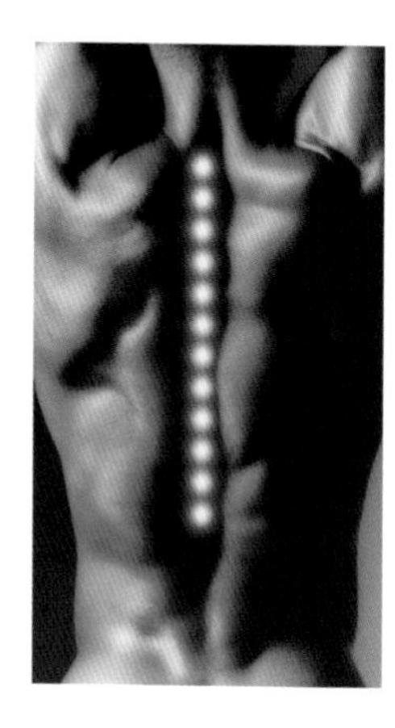

Thoracic spine
The 12 vertebrae of the thoracic spine are firmly attached to the ribs.

Below the vertebrae of the neck are the 12 thoracic vertebrae, extending from the collarbone to just above the waist. The thoracic vertebrae are attached to the ribs. They are larger than the neck vertebrae and, from top to bottom, each one is slightly bigger than the one above it.

The main function of the thoracic vertebrae is to support the rib cage, and because they are anchored by the ribs, they are less prone to wear and tear than the cervical vertebrae. There tend to be fewer problems in this area than in the neck and the lower back.

The ribs, which are linked to your thoracic vertebrae, make a bony cage to protect your vital organs, including your heart, lungs, stomach, spleen, and kidneys. Between each rib space are muscles called intercostals, which lift the ribs upward and outward each time you breathe in, allowing your lungs to expand. When you breathe out, the muscles and the ribs relax again.

Sometimes if you've been coughing a lot, after flu or a chest infection, your ribs can become slightly tilted and too close together. This may also happen after playing sports such as tennis, when constant use of your right arm can affect the rib spaces. You may get a sharp pain in your side—try the exercise on page 80 to ease the pain.

Scoliosis

There are three major deformities that can affect the spine—scoliosis, kyphosis, and lordosis.

Everyone's spine is curved, but in scoliosis the spine also curves from side to side, making an S shape. The condition affects the thoracic spine and the lumbar vertebrae. Symptoms include an obvious curving of the spine, shoulder blades at different heights, and back pain. Some children are born with scoliosis, but most commonly this condition develops in children around the time of puberty. In very severe scoliosis, the rib cage may become affected and heart and breathing problems can follow. Treatment varies according to the severity of the curve. Some sufferers can be treated with orthopedic braces and exercise to prevent further deformity. Other patients need surgery to straighten the crooked spine.

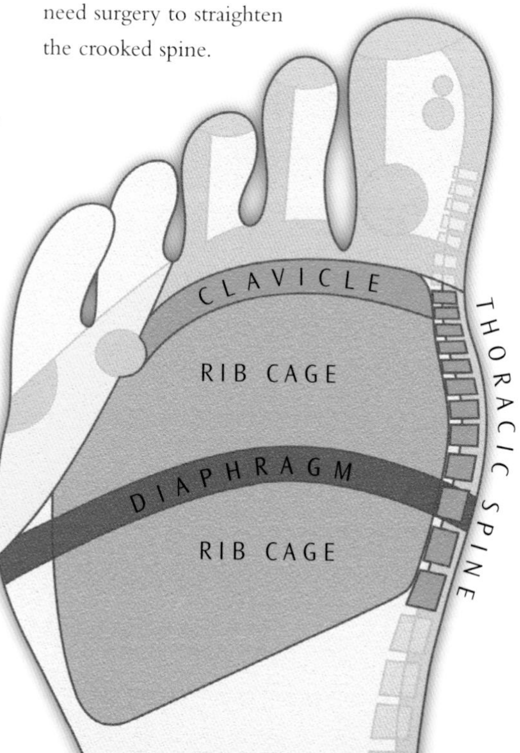

Areas on the foot
The natural curve of the foot echoes the curve of the thoracic spine. For problems with the thoracic spine, work on these reflex points.

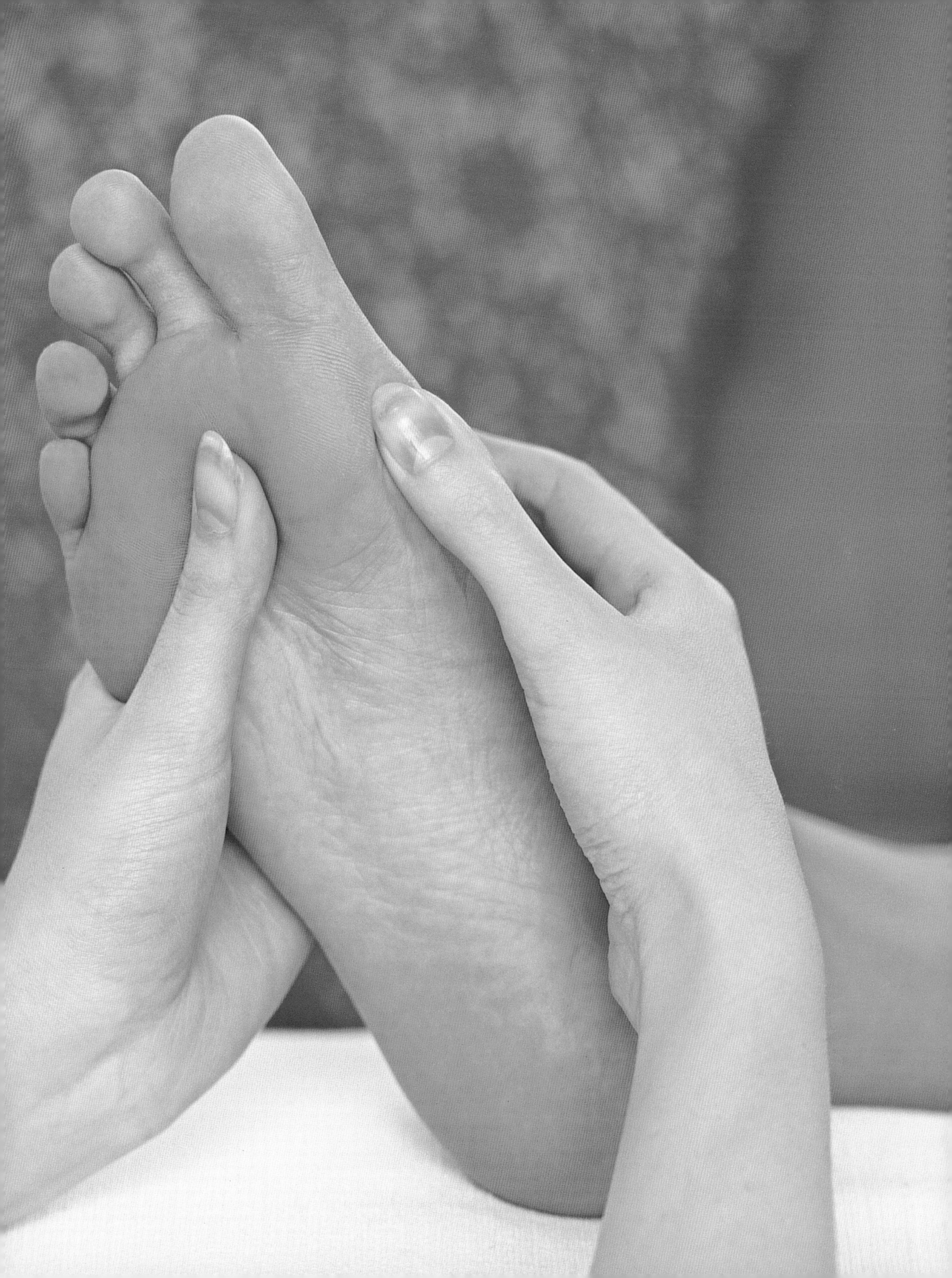

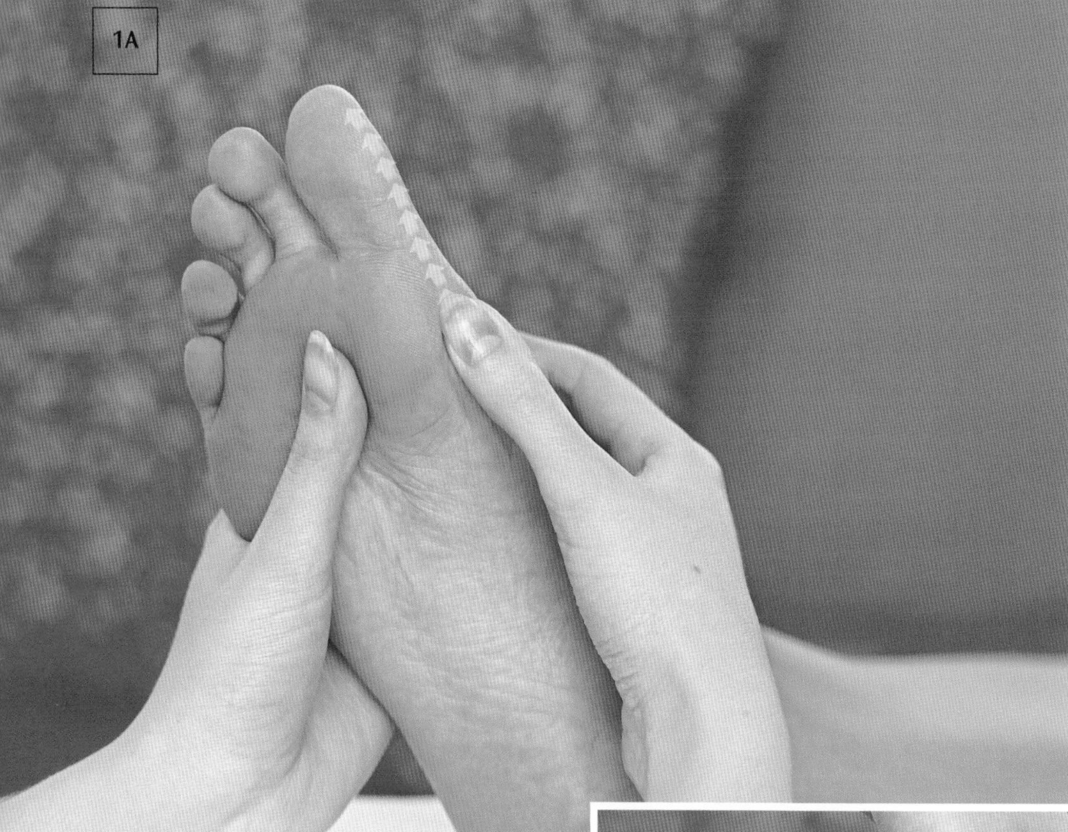

Upper back pain

To treat discomfort in the upper back, support the right foot with the left hand and creep up the inside edge of the foot with the right thumb (1A) and down again with the left thumb (1B). Switch hands to treat the left foot.

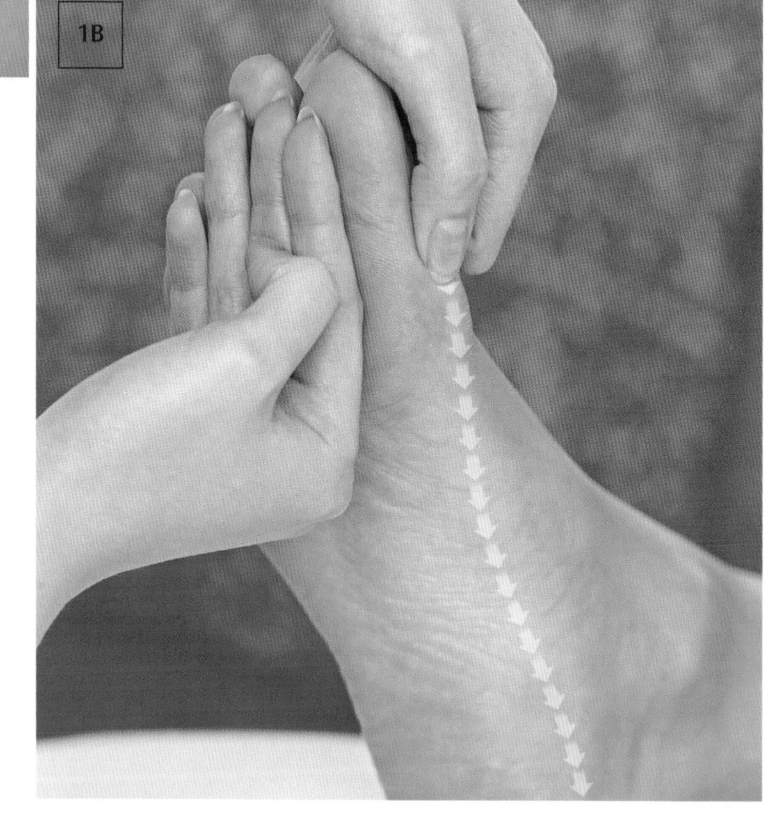

Kyphosis

Kyphosis is an exaggerated rounding of the back and affects the thoracic vertebrae. The spine is hunched over, the shoulders bend forward, and the upper spine has a rounded appearance. The curved area may be painful and reflexology can help ease discomfort. Conditions such as osteoporosis and osteoarthritis are common causes of kyphosis, as are excess weight and poor posture.

Lordosis

Kyphosis can sometimes lead to lordosis because the lower spine is forced to compensate for the greater than usual curve at the top of the spine. In lordosis the lumbar spine curves inward, making the stomach stick out. This is common in late pregnancy, when the enlarged abdomen places extra strain on the spine.

Rib cage

To relax the rib cage and ease pain, press the sole of the right foot with your thumbs (2A). Using the creeping technique, work across the top of the foot with the fingers of both hands (2B, 2C). Repeat on the left foot.

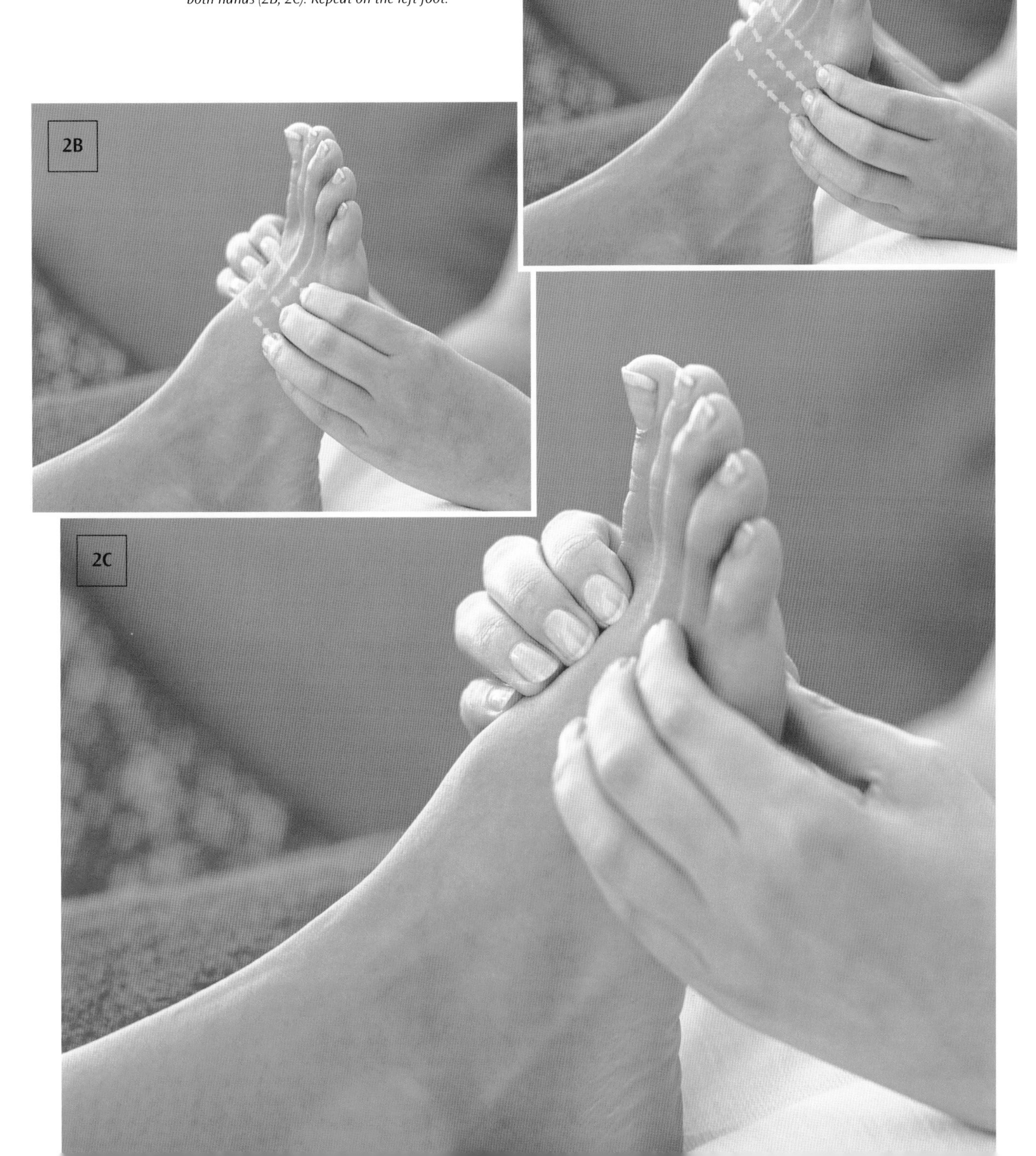

Simple exercises for your upper back

Self traction is a very effective way of easing rib pain, but must be done with great care. Look for a sturdy tree with a good strong branch that can support your weight. Hold the branch tightly, one hand on each side, and lift your feet off the ground for a few seconds. This stretch will separate each of your vertebrae and and will soothe your discomfort. Repeat the exercise several times, but stop immediately if you feel uncomfortable at any time. If you prefer to do this exercise indoors, you can try hanging from a strong door frame or a wall bar in the gym. Whatever you use, always check that it is strong enough to bear your weight.

To help relieve painful spasms in the rib cage, try this breathing exercise which stretches the rib cage. Stand with your arms by your sides. Take as deep a breath in as you can (1), hold for ten seconds (2), then slowly breathe out (3). Repeat several times.

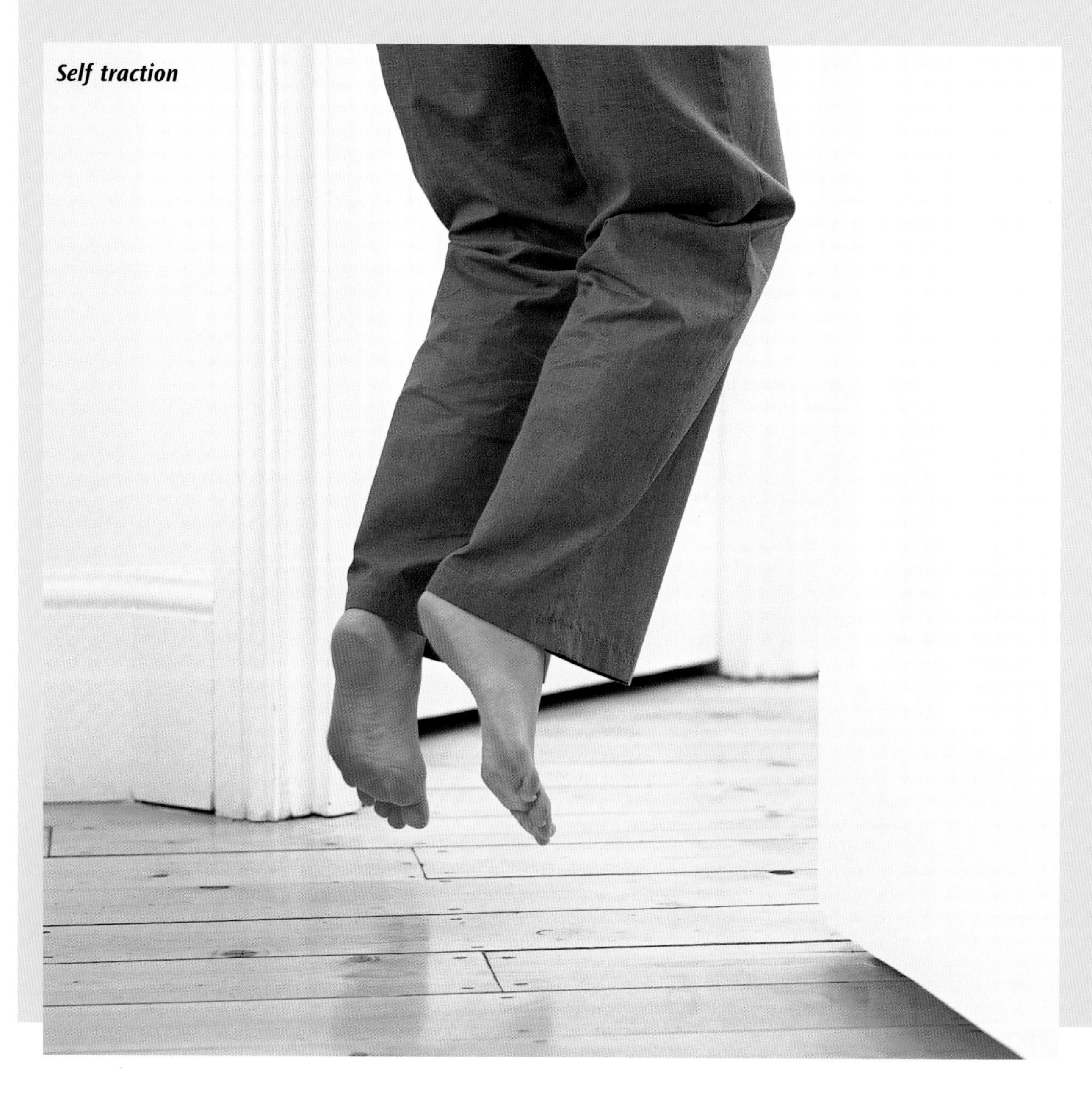

Self traction

Breathing exercise

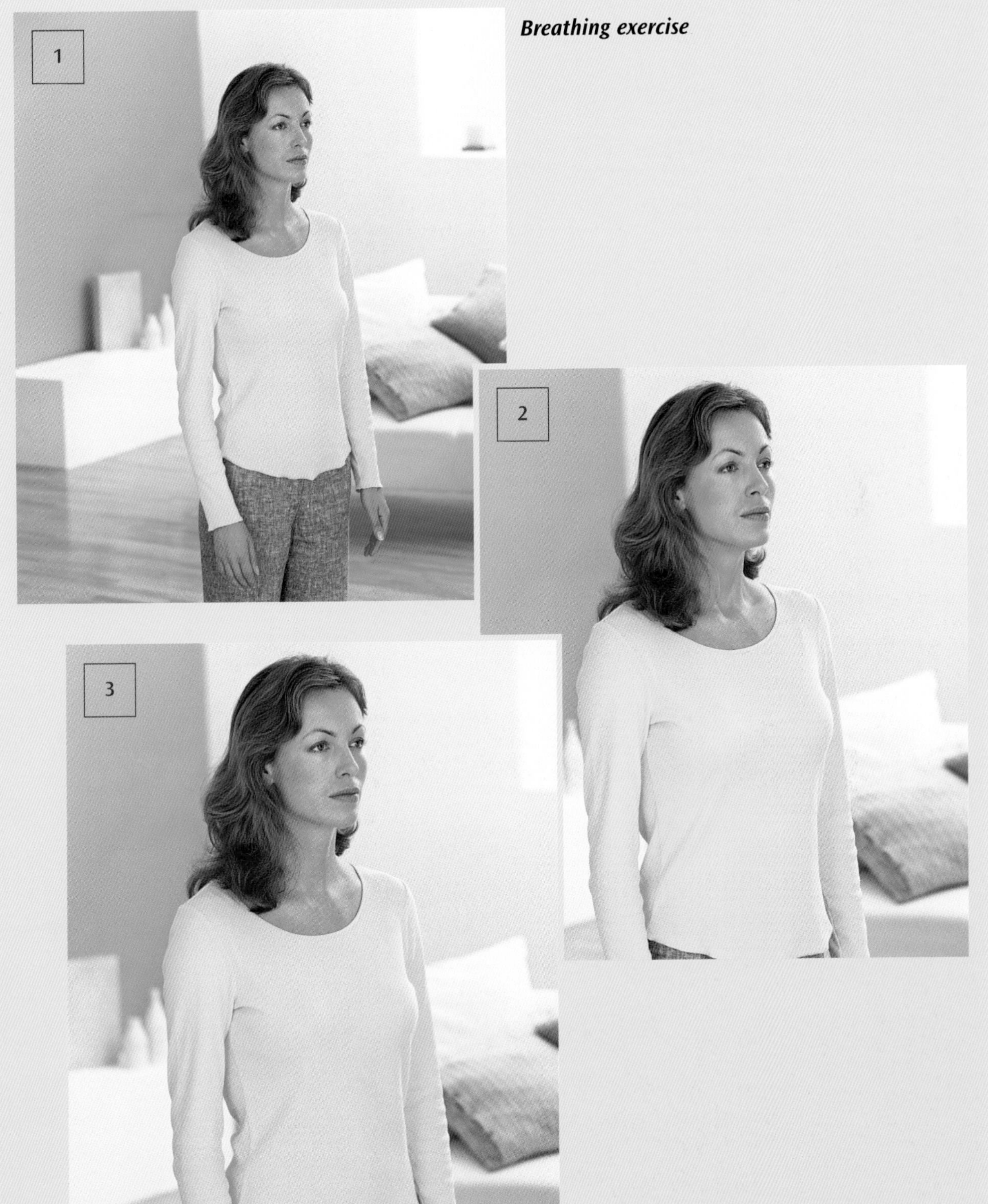

TREATING THE SHOULDER, ARM, & HAND

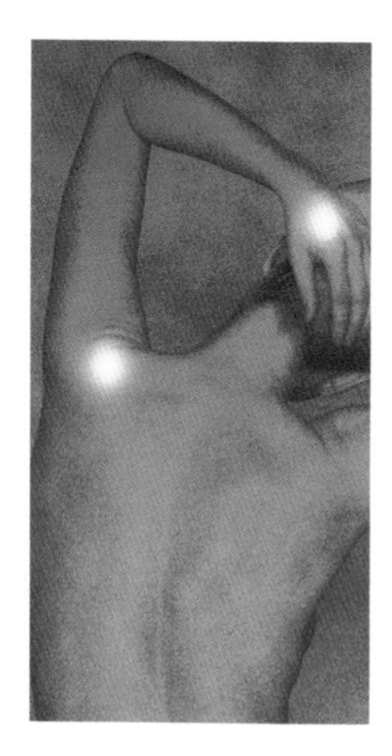

Shoulder, arm, and hand
All these areas can be affected by problems in your neck and spine.

Your shoulders, arms, and hands are very flexible. The shoulder joint allows a far greater range of movement than the hip joint, and the hands are capable of incredibly fine, subtle actions.

Problems in your neck and upper spine can cause pain in your shoulders, arms, and hands. Tingling sensations in your fingers, weakness in your wrists making it difficult to do things such as open jars, and discomfort when lifting your arms above your head so that even combing your hair is an effort, are just a few of the symptoms people have.

The upper arm is linked to the shoulder by a ball and socket joint. Normally, this joint allows the arm to move around in a circle, as well as up and down, forward and backward.

Frozen shoulder

A common problem in this area is frozen shoulder, which can be linked to injury, overuse of the arm, or arthritis in the shoulder. The exact cause is unknown, but there is usually some inflammation of the membrane of the joint which restricts its movement. All joints have a synovial membrane, which is a thin slippery membrane that lines the joint surface. The membrane is filled with a fluid, which helps the joint move smoothly. If there was no membrane on the surface of joints, bone would rub on bone and the joint would soon wear out. When the joint is inflamed, the membrane dries out causing problems. Unfortunately, frozen shoulder can take a long time to heal. Symptoms may last for a year or more, but the shoulder does always get better eventually.

Treating frozen shoulder

An ice pack will help reduce inflammation and ease the pain of a frozen shoulder.

You'll need a pack of frozen peas, a damp wash-cloth, and a small hand towel. Place the washcloth on the painful shoulder, put the frozen peas on top, and cover with the hand towel. Lie face down with the ice pack in place for about 20 minutes. If the shoulder is very painful, repeat the ice pack treatment three or four times a

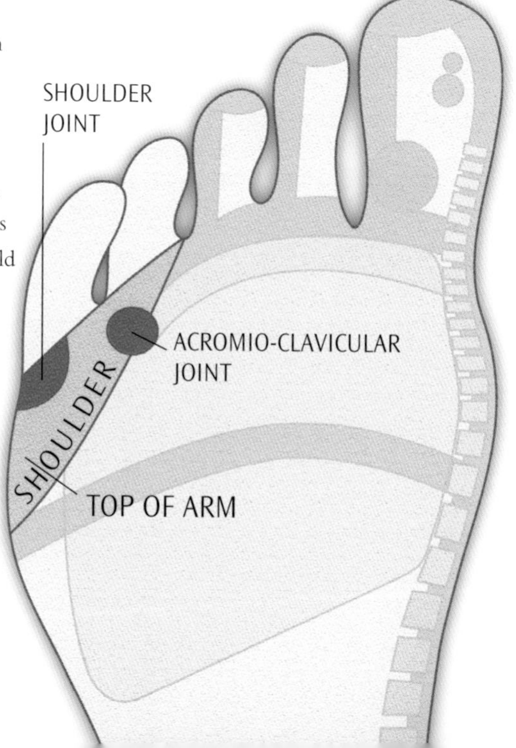

Areas on the foot
For shoulder, arm, and hand problems, concentrate on reflexology points in these areas of the foot.

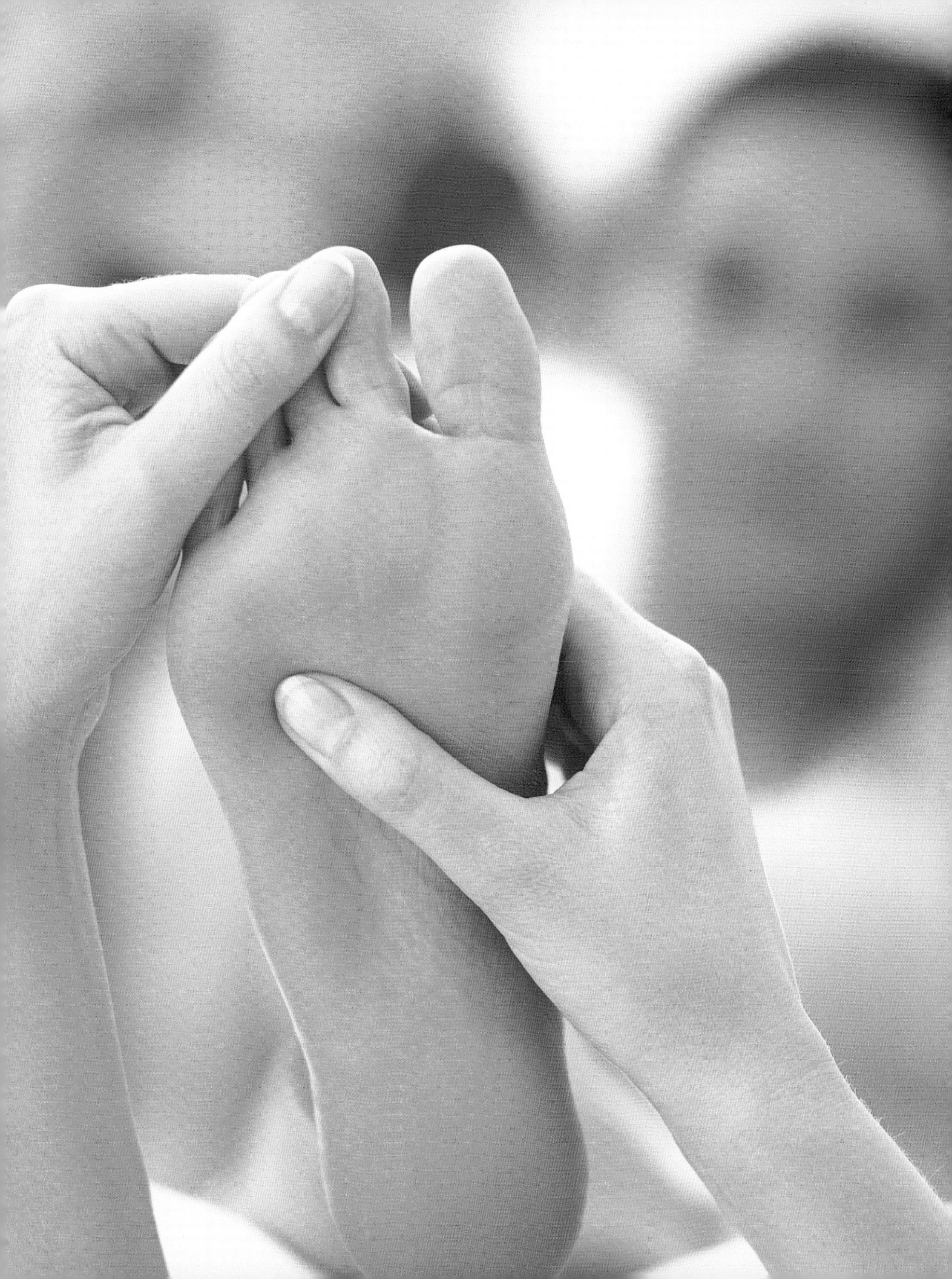

Frozen or arthritic shoulder

Support the top of the right foot with your left hand. Using your right thumb, creep outward across the area below the fourth and fifth toes (1A). Change hands and creep inward with your other thumb (1B). Switch hands to treat the left foot.

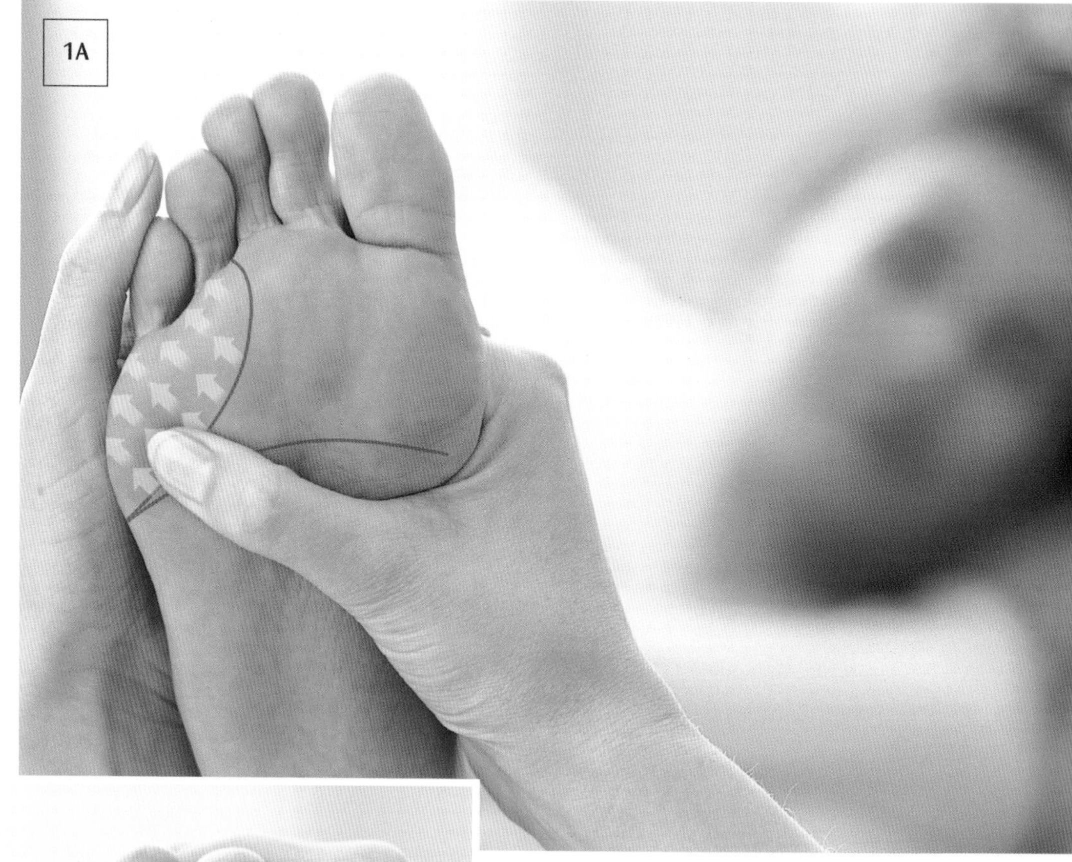

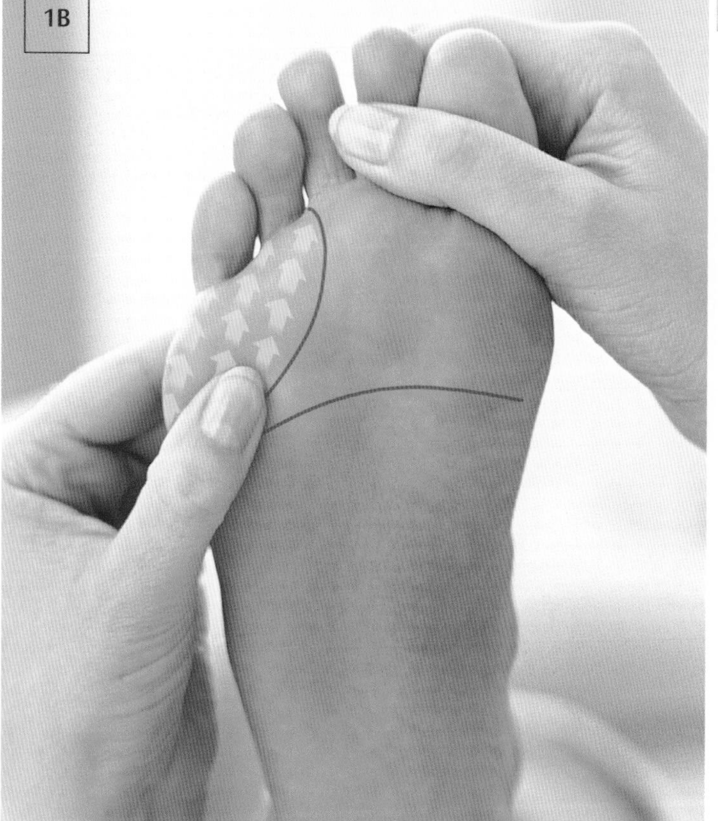

day, remembering to re-freeze the pack of peas each time. Once the shoulder becomes less painful and more mobile, you should start doing some exercises (see pages 88–89). With the help of treatment of the reflexology areas, ice packs, and exercise, your shoulder should soon become pain free and mobile again.

Carpal tunnel syndrome

The carpals are the eight small bones in the wrist, and the carpal tunnel is the space between these bones and the ligament that runs over them. Carpal tunnel syndrome, or repetitive strain injury as it is most commonly known, is a common painful disorder that happens when the median nerve, which runs from the hand into the forearm, becomes compressed or squeezed in the carpal tunnel (see treatment on page 87).

The first symptoms are usually a burning, tingling feeling, particularly in the thumb, index,

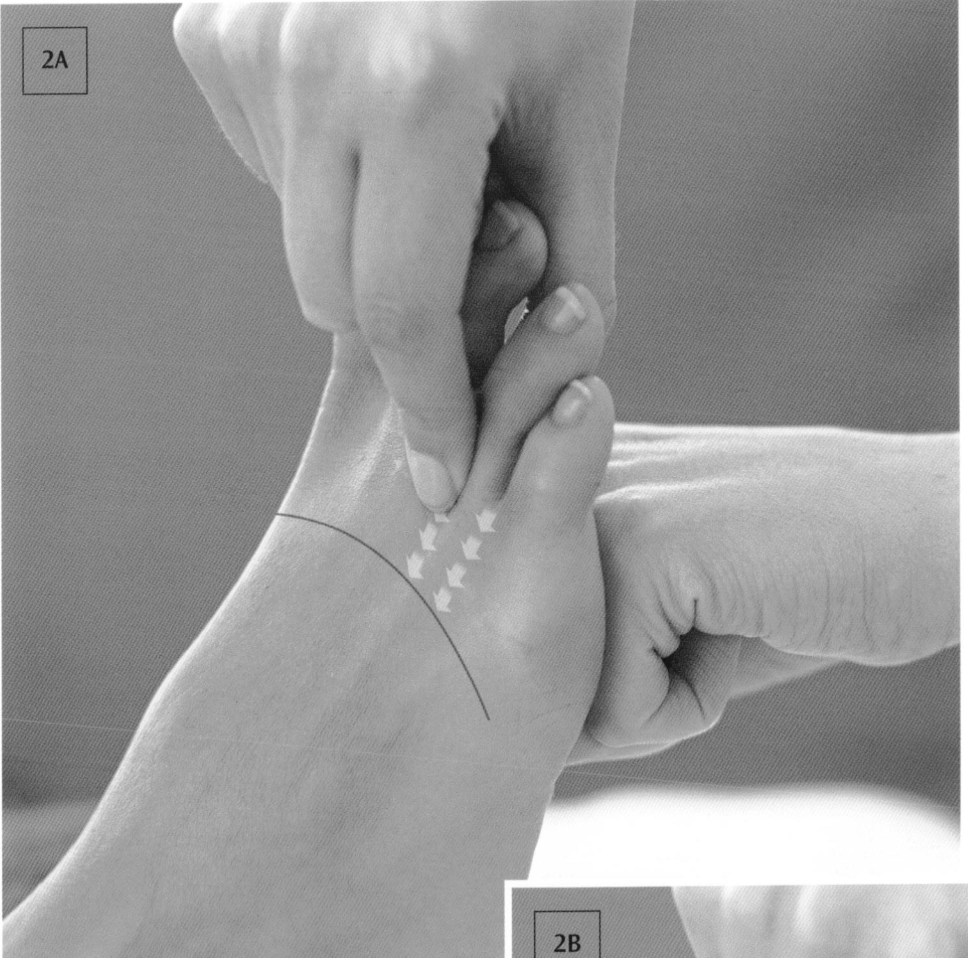
2A

Front of shoulder

Support the right foot against the fist of your left hand. Using your right index finger, creep down the groove between the third and fourth toes (2A).

Continue by creeping down the groove between the fourth and fifth toes (2B). Switch hands to treat the left foot.

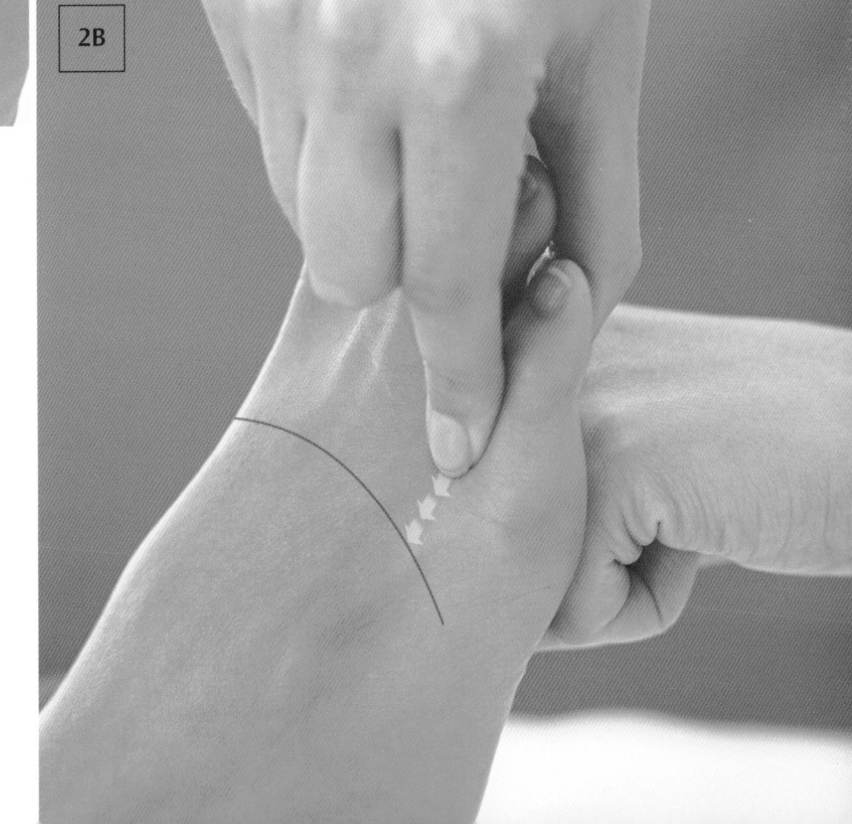
2B

and middle fingers, and in the palm of the hand. It may become hard to make a fist, pick up small things, and perform other tasks with the hands. Symptoms may be felt occasionally or all the time, but are usually worse at night. Women are three times more likely to suffer carpal tunnel syndrome than men.

The condition can have a number of causes but is often the result of doing a repetitive task, such as using a computer keyboard for long periods or assembly line work. Fluid retention can also be a cause and people who have problems with fluid retention often find a low-salt diet helpful. Too much salt and too many refined carbohydrates can build up fluid in the tissue spaces and contribute

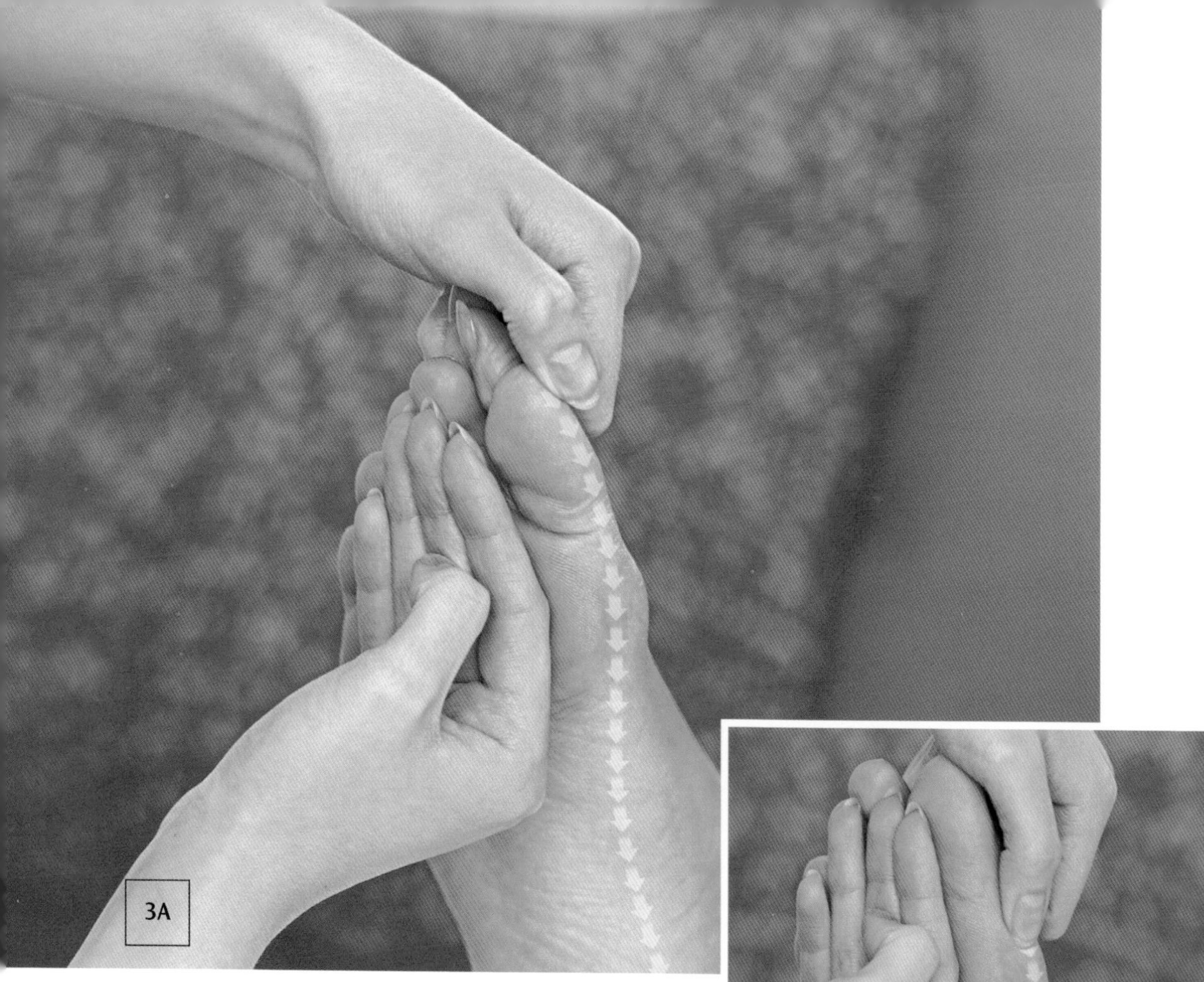

to the congestion of the nerves in the wrist. Sometimes it follows injuries to the wrist, but this is not the norm.

Carpal tunnel syndrome is common in pregnant women because the hormonal changes, in particular high levels of estrogen, create more fluid in the tissues. The fluctuating hormonal surges women experience during menopause can give rise to the same symptoms.

Easing symptoms

Vitamin B6 deficiency has been found to be an underlying cause of carpal tunnel syndrome and sufferers really need ten times the usual recommended daily allowance.

Turmeric (also known as Indian saffron) has been used in both the Indian (Ayurvedic) and Chinese systems of medicine for treating

Spine (down)

Working the upper spine in both directions can help shoulder pain, as nerves arising fom the entire spine have a great effect in relieving tension. Support the right foot with the back of your right hand. Use your left thumb to creep down the inside edge of the foot (3A, 3B, 3C). Switch hands to treat the left foot.

many forms of inflammation. The volatile oil in the spice has been demonstrated in a variety of studies to have anti-inflammatory properties. Ice pack treatment (see pages 82–84) can also be helpful.

Preventing carpal tunnel syndrome

If you're at risk for carpal tunnel syndrome, it may help to do stretching exercises at work and take regular breaks to rest your wrists and hands. Some people find wearing splints on the wrists or using wrist supports when typing helpful. Always try to make sure that computers and any other equipment you use is correctly positioned. Keeping the hands warm while you're working is also said to help, so try wearing fingerless gloves.

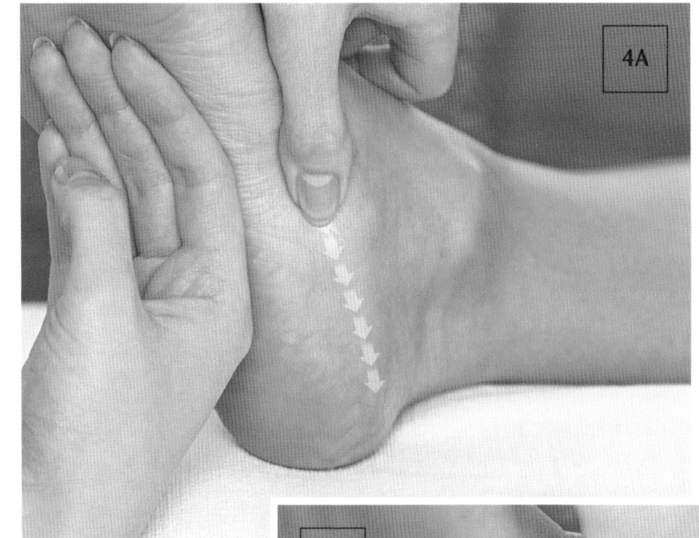

Spine (down)

Supporting the heel of the right hand in the palm of your right hand, work down the medial edge of the foot to the base of the heel (4A, 4B). Switch hands to treat the left foot.

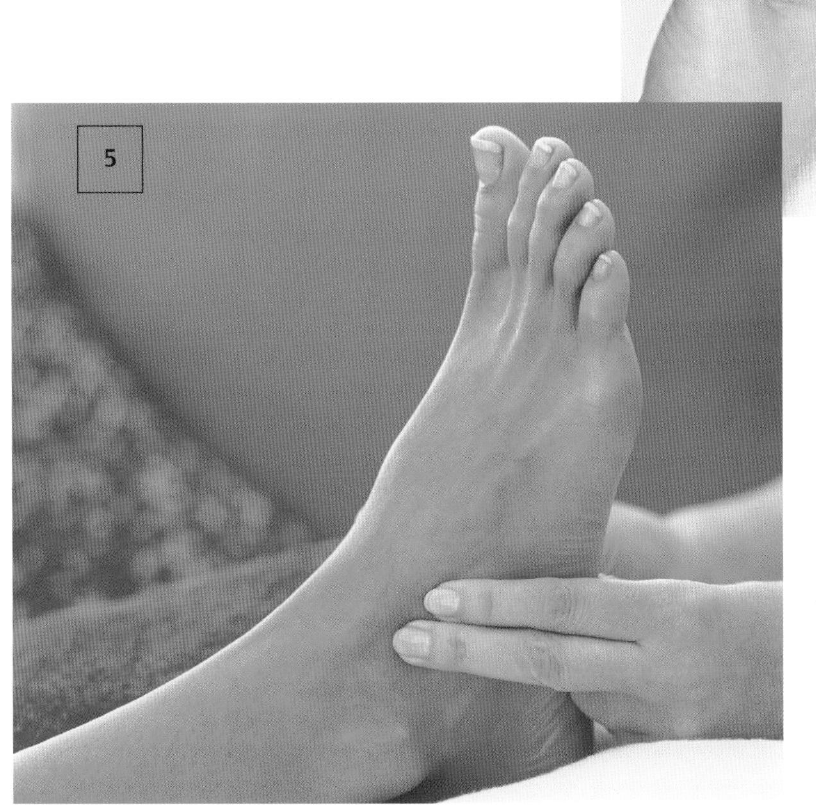

Wrist—carpal tunnel syndrome

This area at the top of the foot contains the reflex points for the wrist. Hold the right foot and press the sole with both thumbs. With the index and third fingers of both hands, creep across the top of the foot two or three times (5). Repeat on the left foot.

Simple shoulder exercises

Once a frozen shoulder starts to become less painful and more mobile, it will really help to start doing arm-walking exercises. Stand facing a wall—get as close as you can. Starting at about waist level, walk your fingers up the wall until eventually you can get your arm above the level of your head (1, 2, 3).

Another good exercise is to try to hold your arms out to your sides (4), bring them in front of you (5) and then extend them backward (6). You'll need to persevere with these exercises for a few days before you'll be able to do them effectively, but the results will be worth the effort.

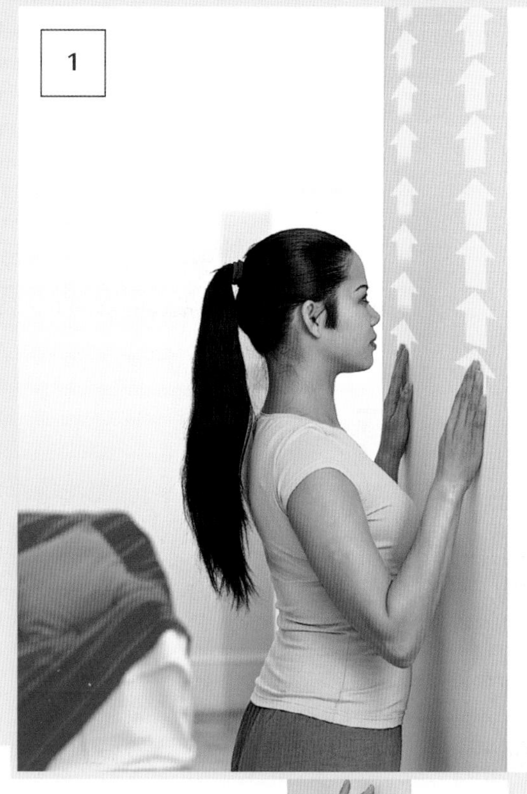

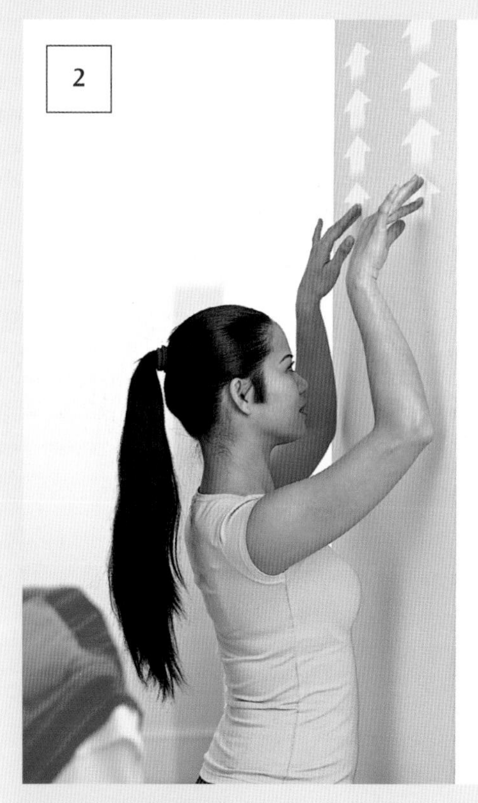

Arm walking

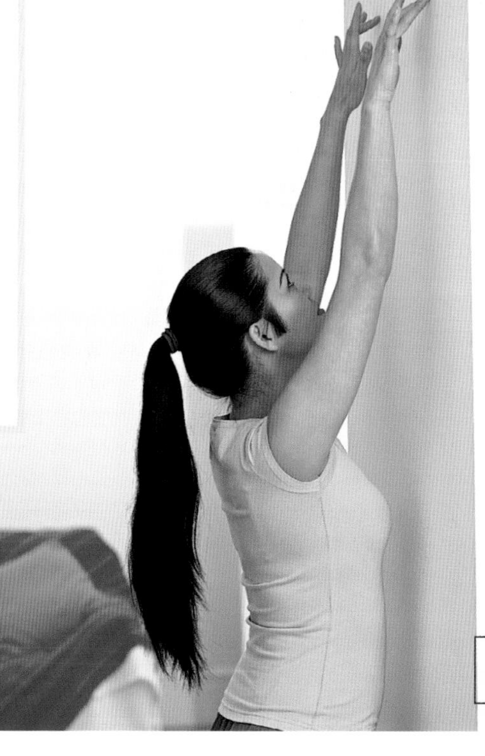

Shoulder rotation

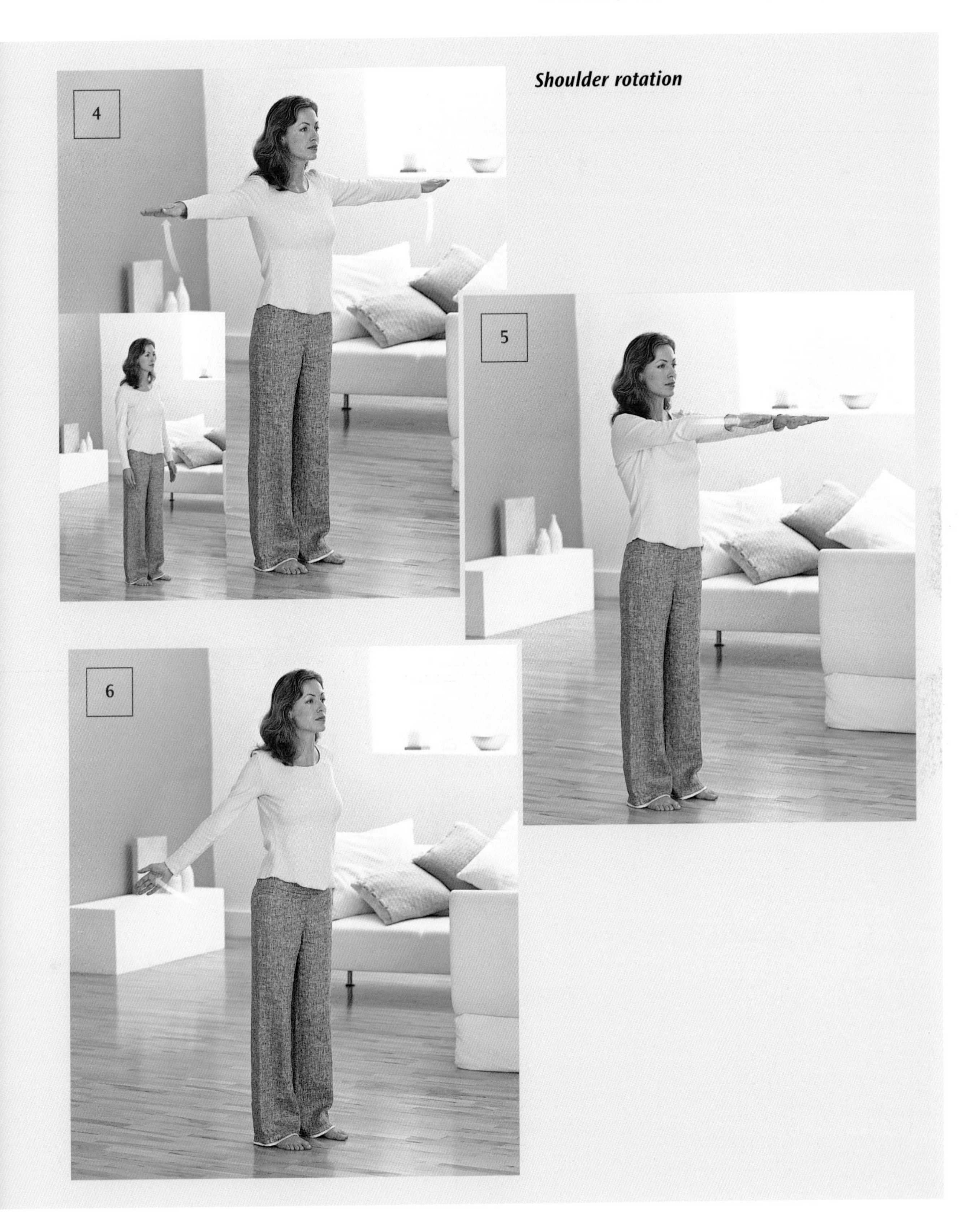

TREATING THE LOWER BACK

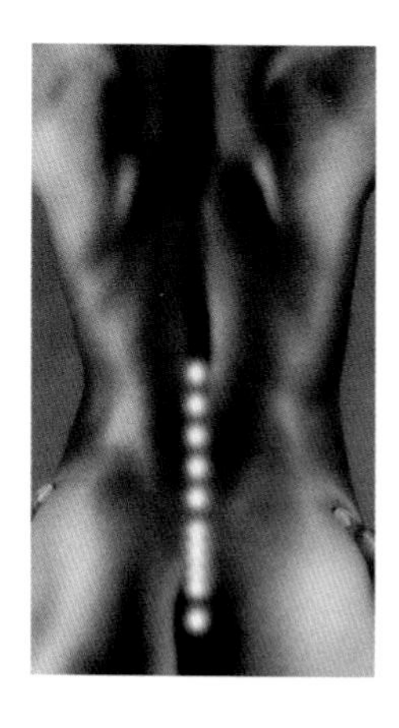

The lower back
The five lumbar vertebrae are stronger and denser than the cervical and thoracic vertebrae. This strength is important—it allows you to stand up, to walk, and to lift.

The lower spine is made up of the five lumbar vertebrae. These are the largest of all the vertebrae—they need to be because they have to bear most of the body's weight. Below these are the five fused bones of the sacrum, which acts as an anchor to the base of the spine. At the bottom of the sacrum is the tailbone or coccyx. This is all that is left of the tail we would have had when we walked on all fours. The lower spine area causes more pain and problems, and is the reason for more sick days off from work, than any other part of the back. Lumbago, sciatica, and prolapsed discs are all related to problems in the lumbar spine.

The lumbar spine twists and bends to permit a range of movement unequalled by any machine. Equipped with highly sophisticated shock absorbers and a remarkable lubrication system, the living human skeleton is also more durable than any man-made creation.

Lower back pain can have a number of causes, including muscle strain, arthritis (see page 12), and osteoporosis (see pages 106–109). Being overweight and smoking can also damage the lower back. To keep your lower back healthy, exercise regularly, take care when lifting heavy loads, keep your weight down, and watch your posture (see page 15).

Keeping cartilage healthy

If you have a lower back problem, it's common to wake up feeling stiff and tense. The more pain you have, the less likely you are to want to exercise, and so the problem gets worse.

The reason for this stiffness is very often the deterioration of the soft cartilage that covers the ends of bones where they meet at joints. You'll probably have noticed this tough, bendy, elastic substance when you're eating a wing or leg of chicken. For your joints to remain healthy, it's essential that the cartilage—which protects your bones against the thousands of mini-shocks caused by each and every one of your movements—retains its elasticity. Supple, strong cartilage allows the ends of bones to rub against each other without causing damage. Joint cartilage holds water that helps the surfaces move smoothly over

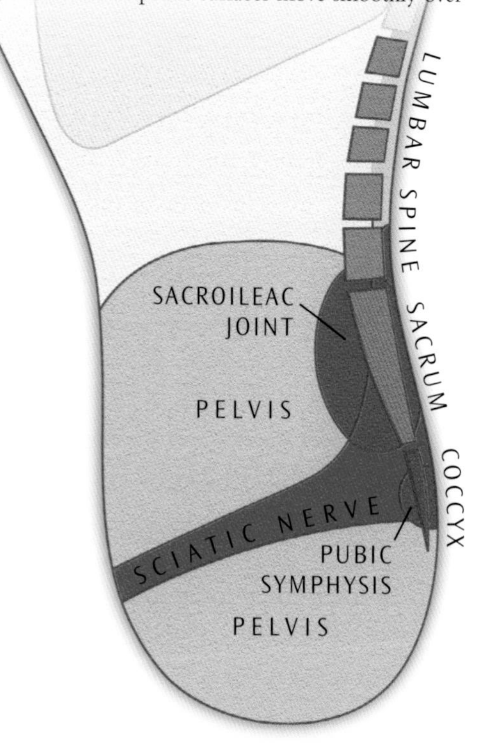

Areas on the foot
For the lower back, concentrate reflexology treatment on these areas.

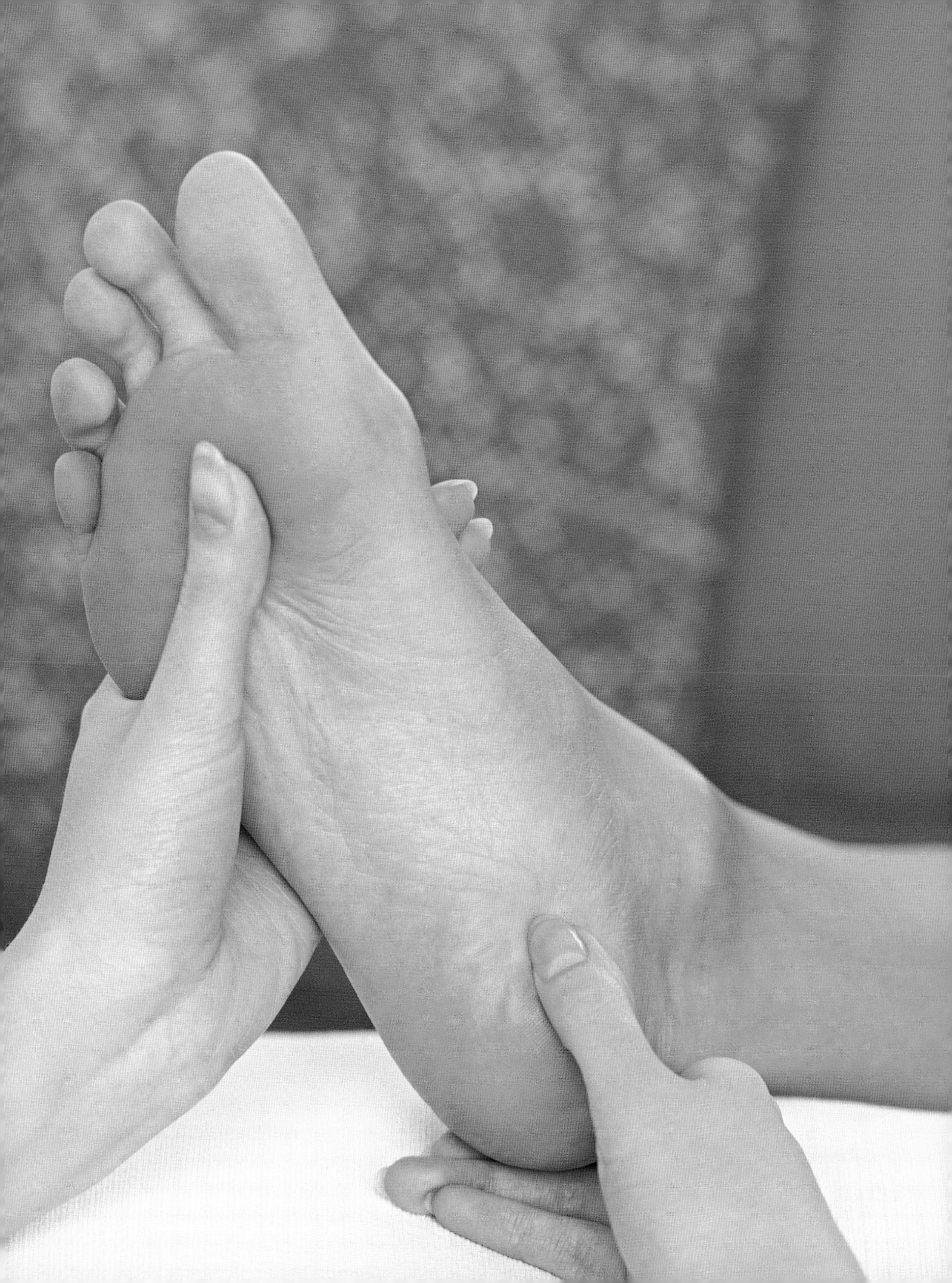

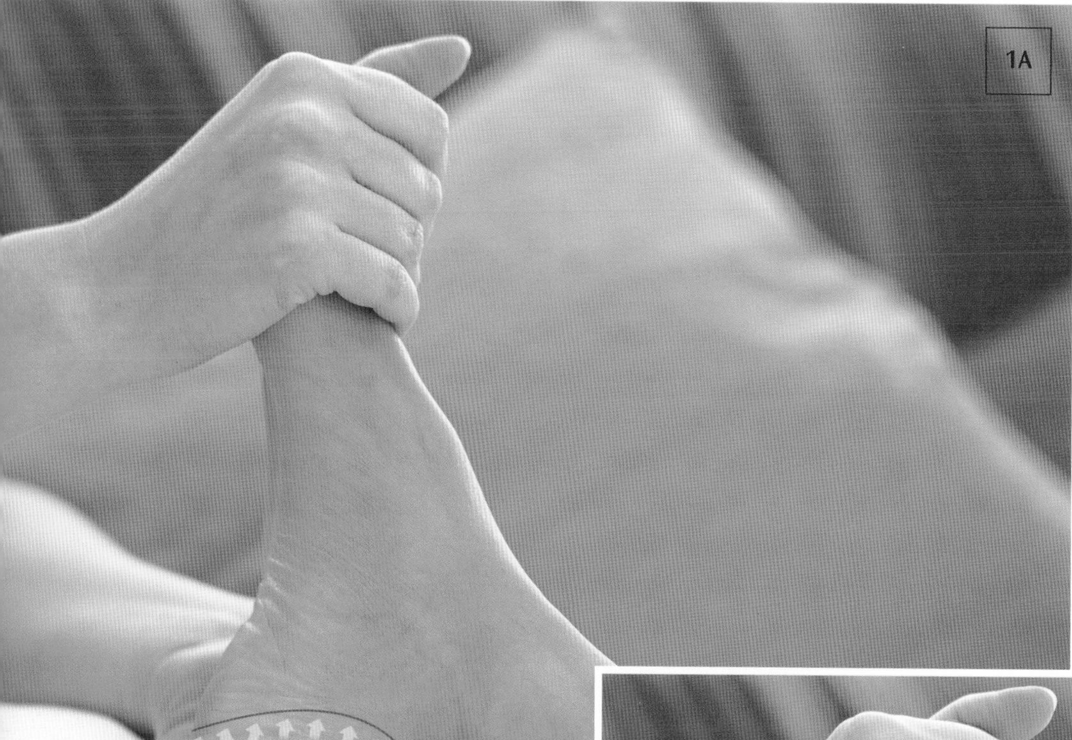

Coccyx

To treat coccyx problems, hold the right foot at the top with your right hand. Using the four fingers of your left hand, creep up the inside of the heel (1A, 1B). Switch hands to treat the left foot.

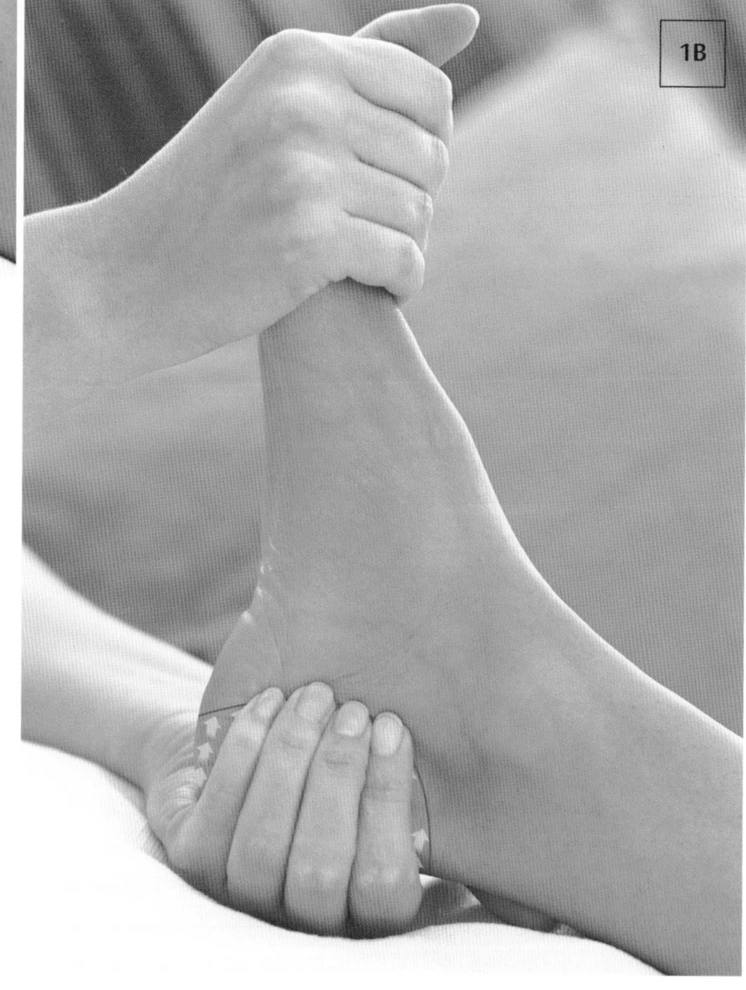

one another when the joint moves. Well-hydrated joints are better able to support the weight of the body and move more easily. If joints become dehydrated, there's more friction in the joint—the cartilage deteriorates and there's damage and pain. Anyone suffering lower back pain should increase their water intake and cut down or cut out dehydrating drinks, including coffee and alcohol.

Strong muscles

It's also important to keep muscles strong so that they can support the vertebral column, buttocks, and abdomen. Indeed, weak abdominal muscles are often the cause of a weakened lower back. It's all too common these days to see men with a lot of weight in front—a beer belly. This extra weight is a constant dragging pressure on the lower back

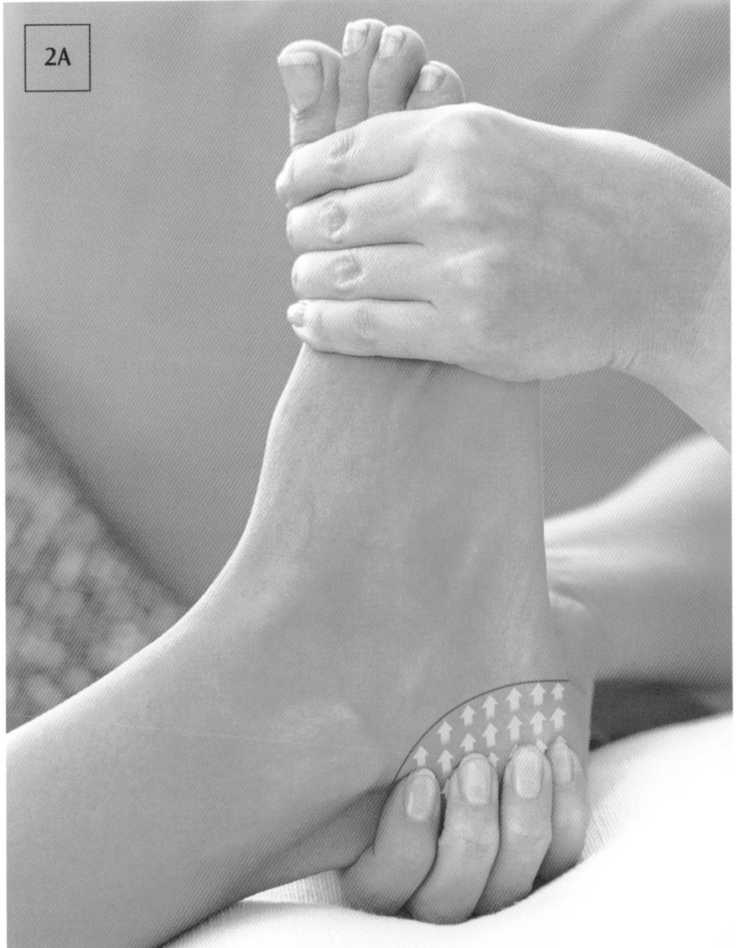

and can lead not only to very bad posture, but also to a painful and very stressed lumbar spine.

Sciatica

Sciatica is one of the most excruciating pains anyone can experience. An attack of sciatica can confine you to bed, with even the slightest movement causing pain.

The sciatic nerves are the largest nerves in the body. Each one is the size of your little finger—most nerves are as thin as the hair on your head. The sciatic nerve is the major nerve of the leg and runs from the lower back down the back of each leg. Above the knee joint the nerve divides into two main branches—the tibial and common peroneal nerves—which extend down the lower legs to the feet.

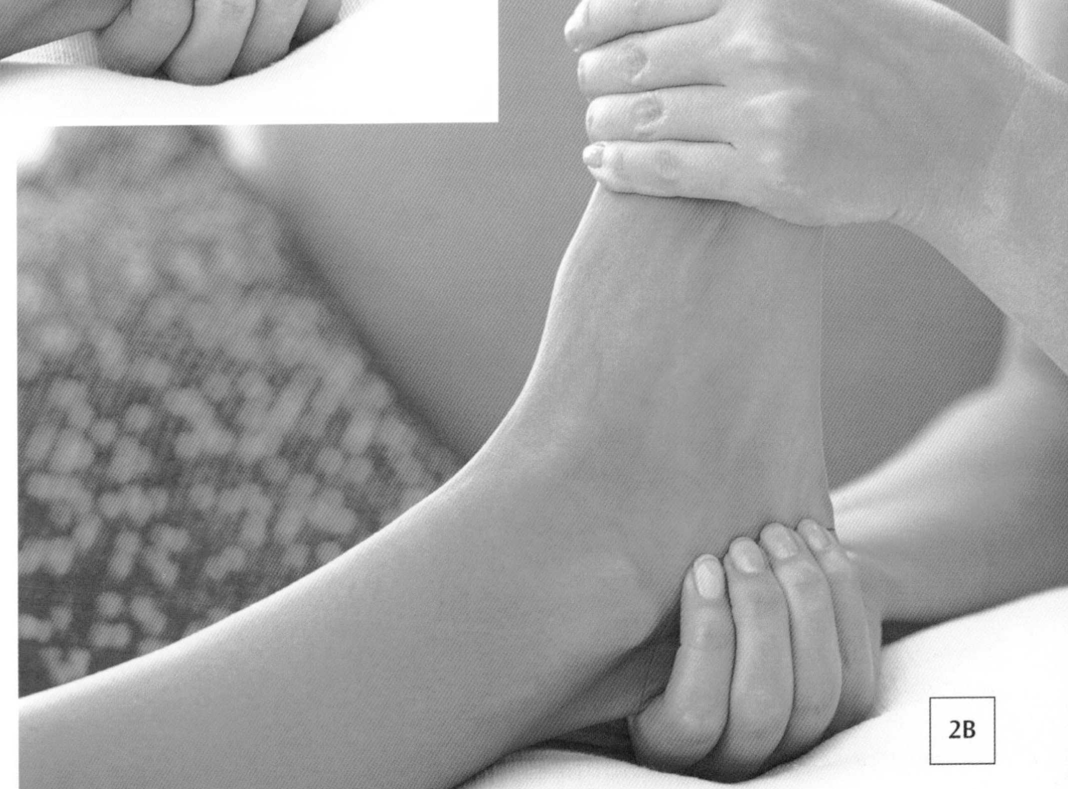

Hip and pelvis

To treat the hip and pelvic problems such as an arthritic hip, hold the right foot with your left hand and work the outside of the heel with your right hand (2A, 2B). Switch hands to treat the left foot.

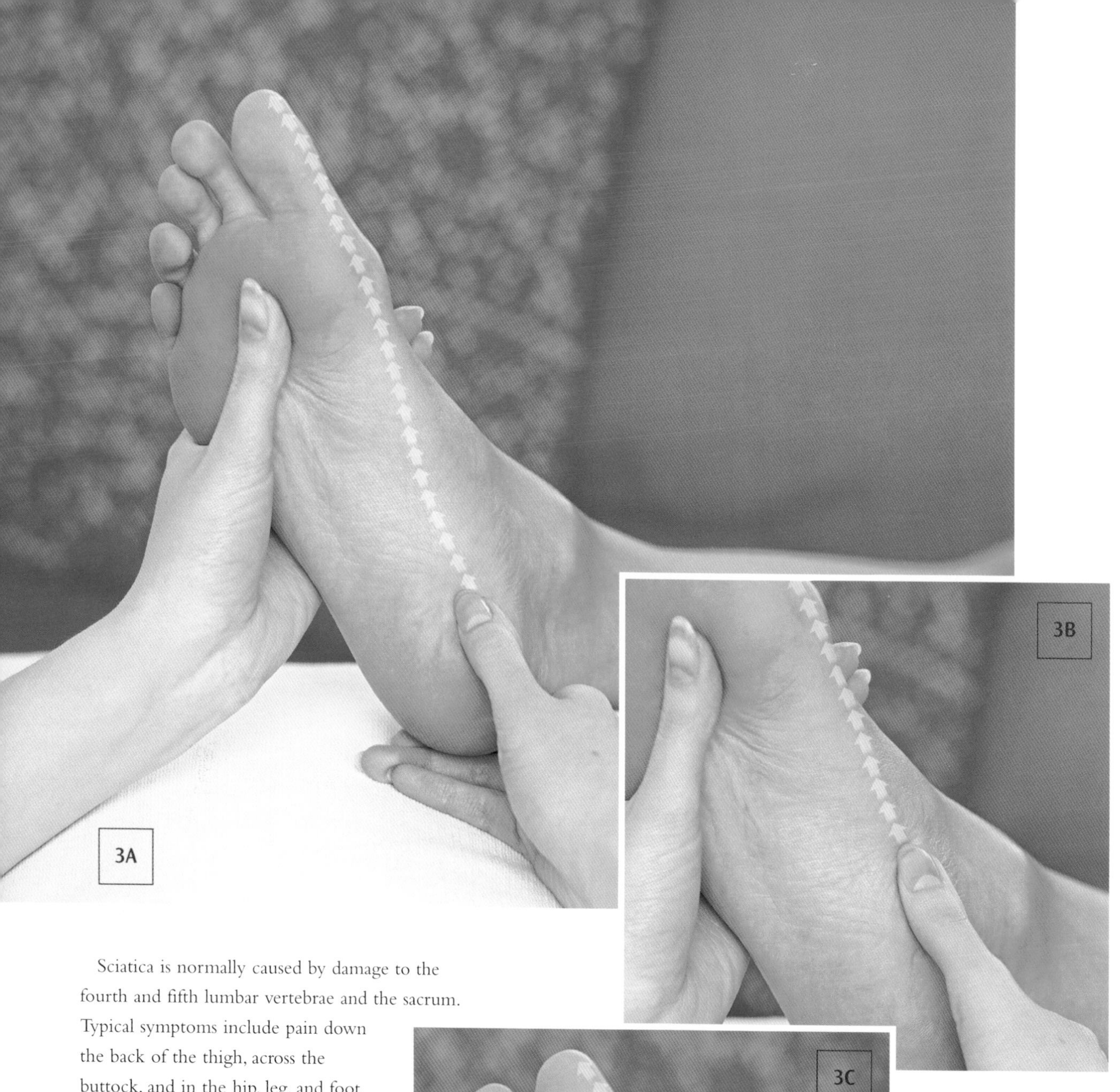

Sciatica is normally caused by damage to the fourth and fifth lumbar vertebrae and the sacrum. Typical symptoms include pain down the back of the thigh, across the buttock, and in the hip, leg, and foot. It's usually impossible to raise the leg off the bed for more than a few inches, and some people are unable to stand.

The most common reason for sciatic pain is a herniated disc. This happens when the core of a disc pushes outward and ruptures, causing swelling and inflammation that presses on the sciatic nerve. A disc prolapse can happen suddenly, brought on by lifting something heavy.

Sciatica is also common in pregnancy when the extra weight at the front of

Spine (up)

To treat pain in the lumbar area, such as disc problems and muscle strain, work up, then down the spine. Support the right foot with your left hand. Creep up the inside edge of the foot with your thumb (3A, 3B, 3C). Work up to the big toe. Repeat on the left foot, using your left thumb.

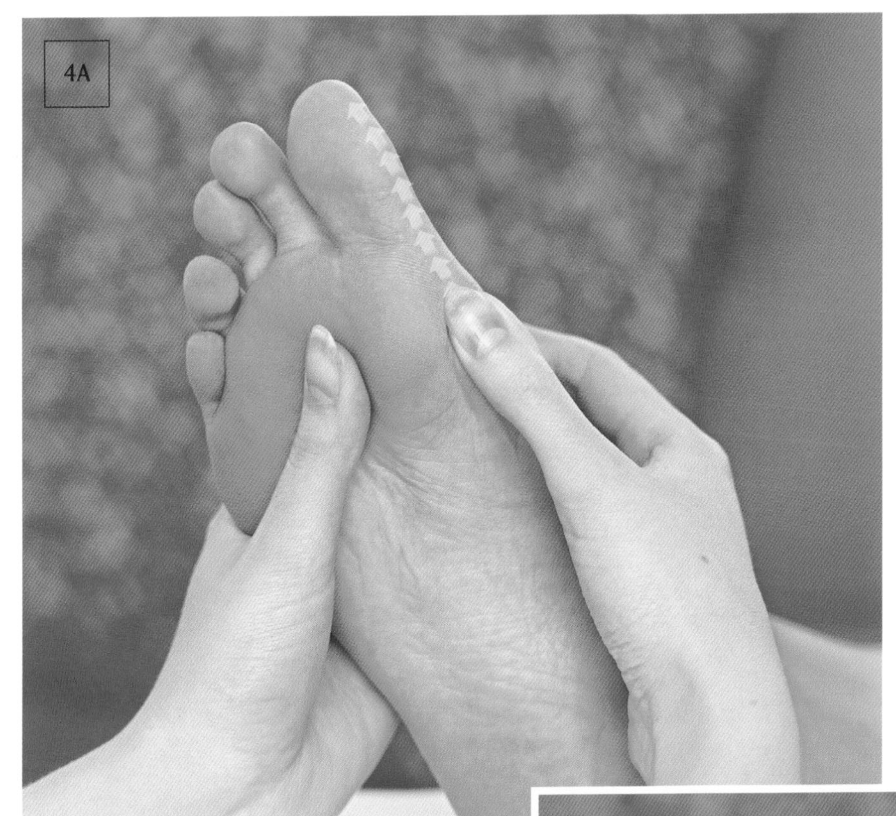

Spine (up)

This treatment helps all back conditions. Support the right foot with the left hand. Work up the entire inside edge of the foot with the right thumb (4A, 4B). Switch hands to treat the left foot.

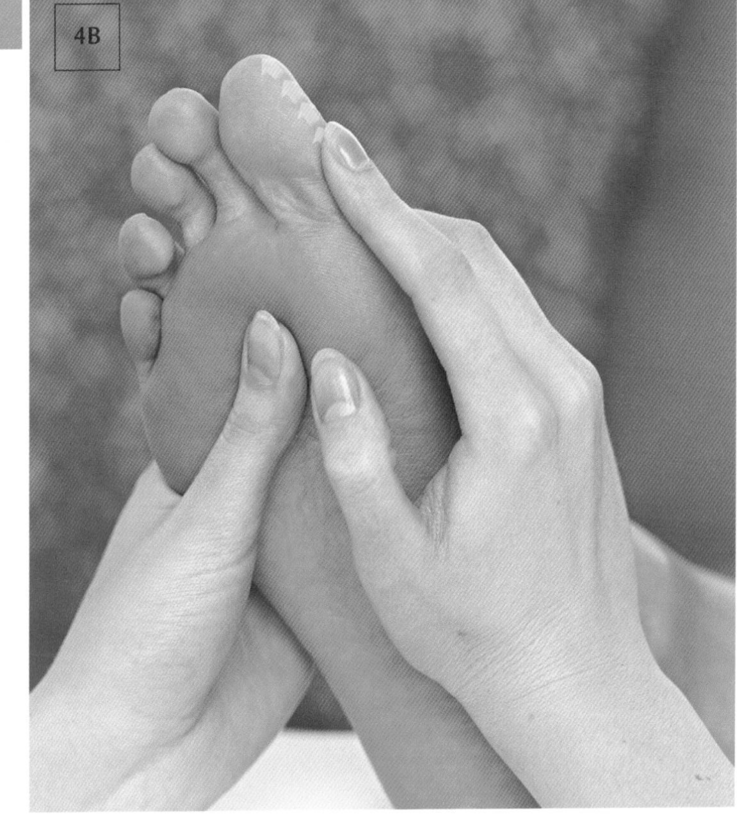

the body can put pressure on the sciatic nerve, and in old age, because of changes in the spine due to arthritis and other conditions. Sciatica that starts during pregnancy usually disappears once the baby is born.

Usually only one leg is affected. The pain may last for a couple of weeks, but may recur.

Treating sciatica

Reflexology has proved very effective in treating sciatica. Other self-help measures include bed rest on a firm mattress and gentle exercise. It's a good idea to place a pillow between your knees when you lie on your side as you sleep; this helps to take the pressure off the sciatic nerve.

Ice packs are recommended for any inflamed area so try this treatment, too (see page 82). And avoid all alcohol, sugar, and high protein foods while suffering from sciatica. These foods cause an acidic condition of the blood, which increases pain.

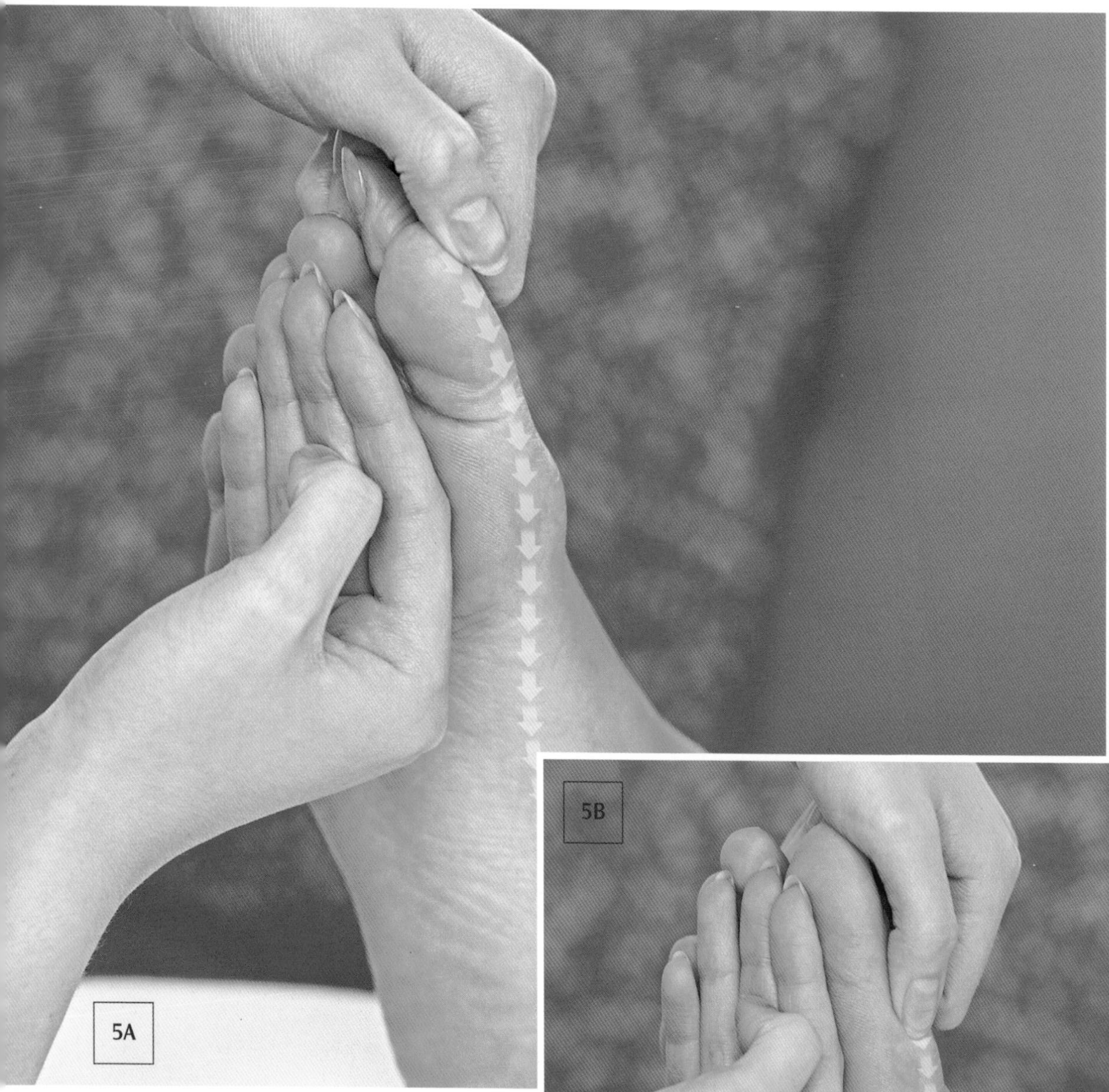

5A

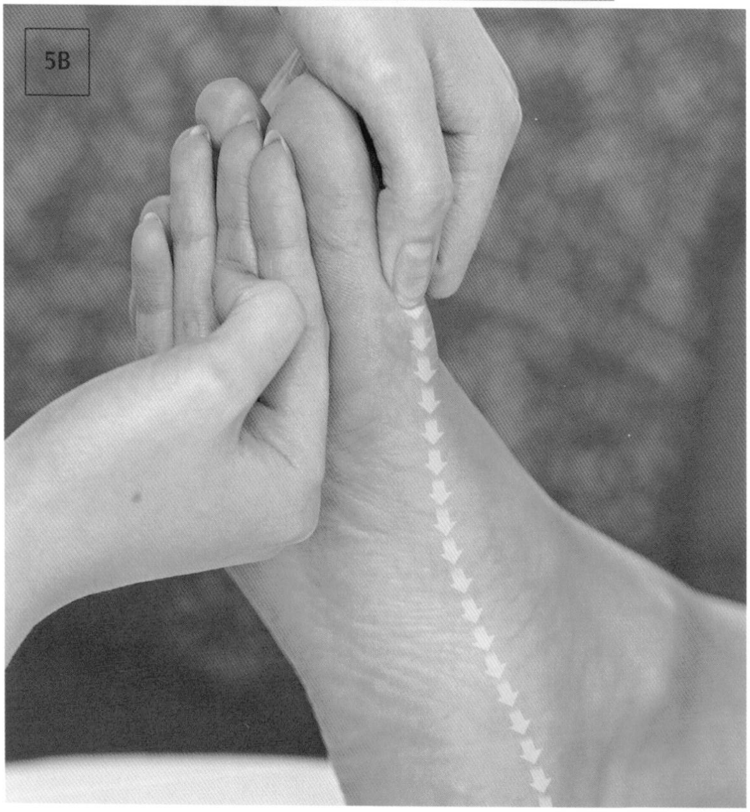

5B

Spine (down)

Support the sole of the right foot with the back of your right hand. Using your left thumb, slowly creep down the inside edge of the foot (5A, 5B).

Spine (down)

Continue working down the foot with your thumb, moving your supporting hand down as you go (5C, 5D, 5E). Switch hands to treat the left foot.

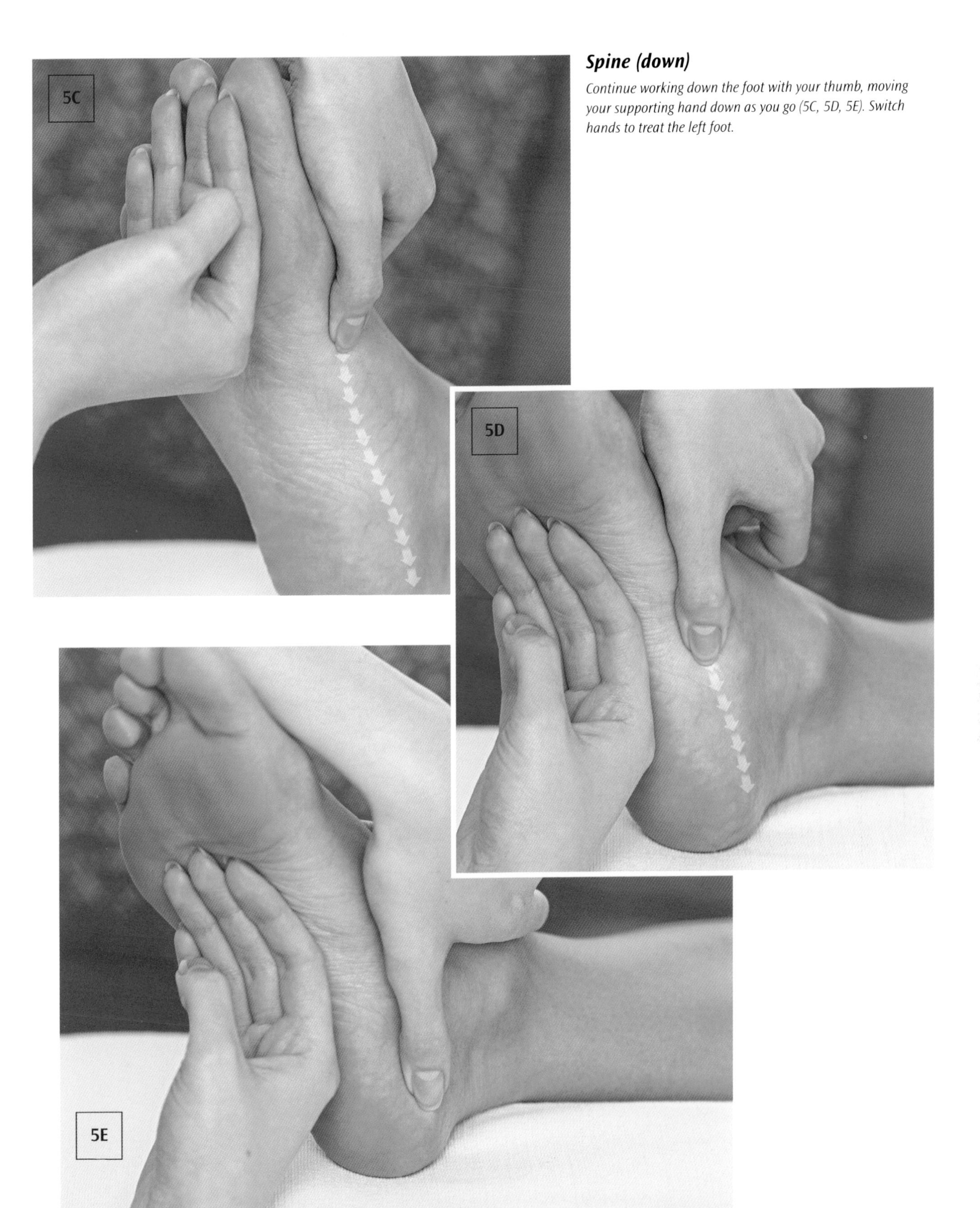

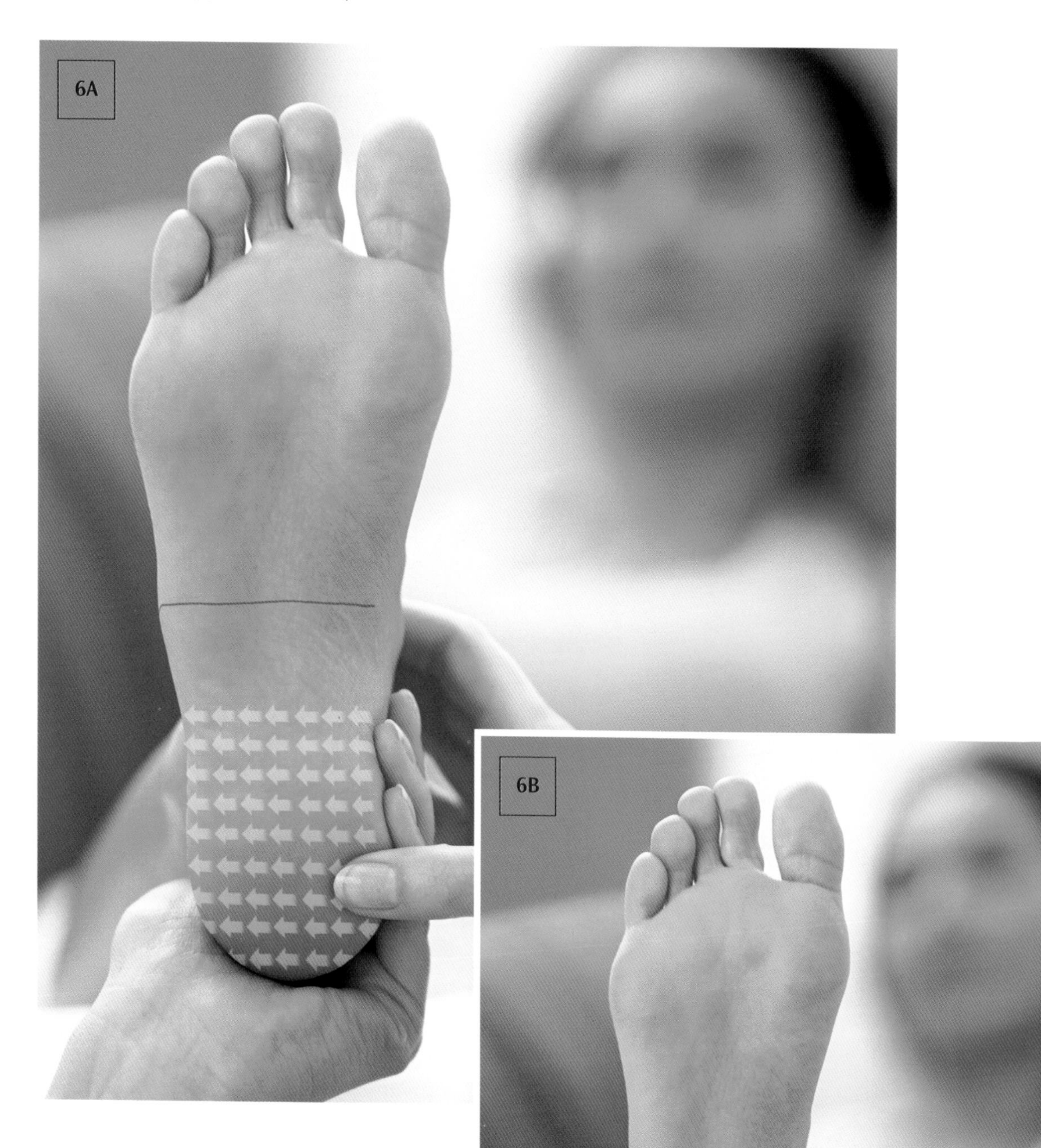

Hip and back of pelvis

Support the heel of the right foot in the palm of the left hand. With the right thumb, work across the base of the heel to contact the sciatic nerve and buttock area (6A). Change hands and work back across the heel (6B). Work the left foot, starting by holding the foot in the right hand and working across with the left thumb.

Primary sciatic

Support the top of the right foot with your right hand. Using your left index finger, creep up the area behind the ankle bone (7A). Continue creeping up the ankle for about 1½ inches (4 cm) (7B). Switch hands to treat the left foot.

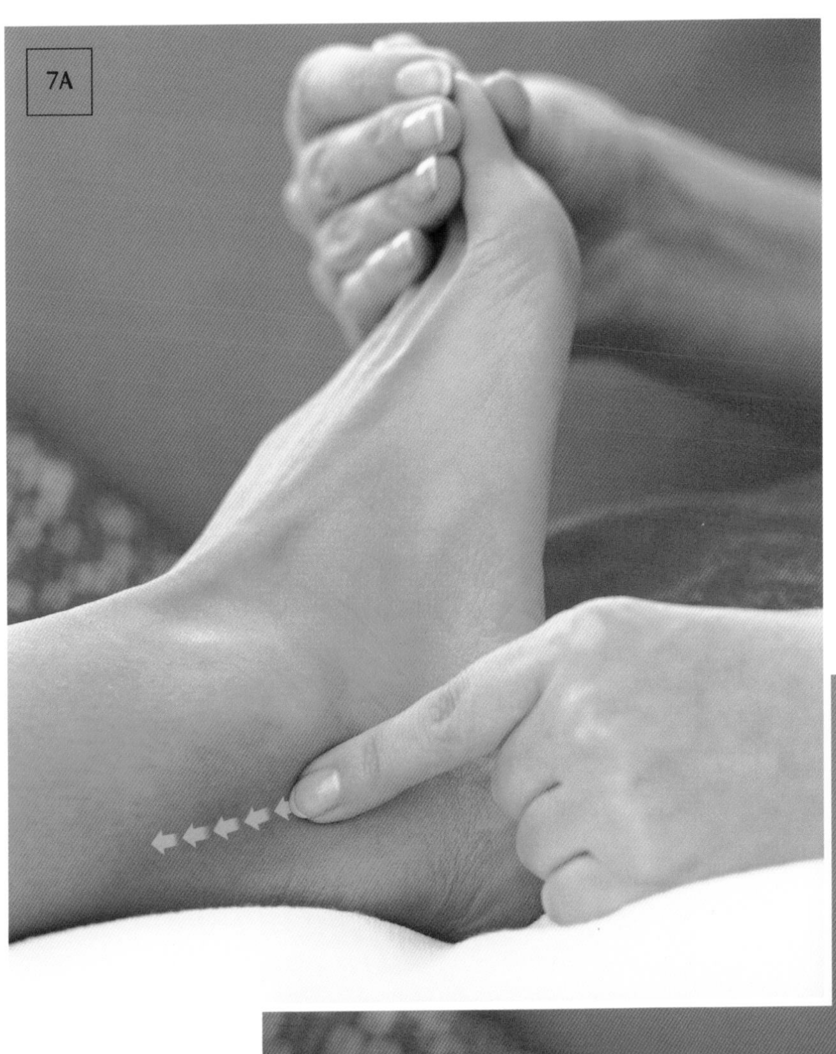
7A

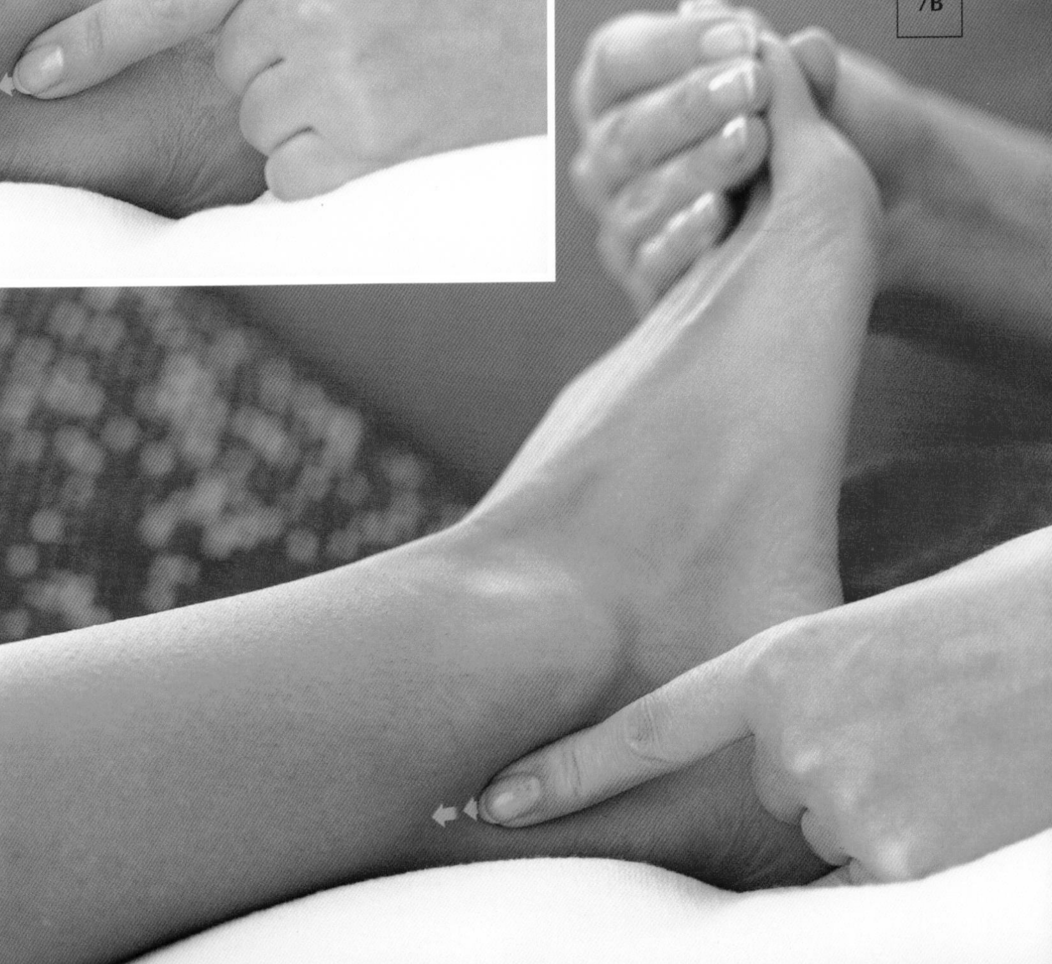
7B

Secondary sciatic

The secondary sciatic point lies across the heel, about halfway between the bottom of the foot and the pelvic line. Using your thumb, creep along this line from the medial side of the right foot to the lateral side. Repeat two or three times (8). Repeat on the left foot.

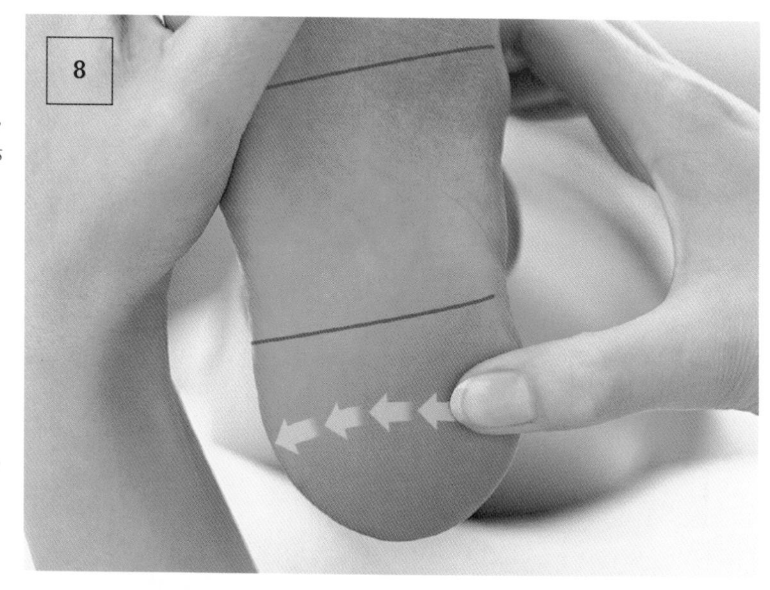

Spinal stimulation point

This reflex point energizes the entire spine. It can be found in the middle of the medial side of the foot. Using your thumb make five or six firm rotations at this point (9) on the right foot. Repeat on the left foot.

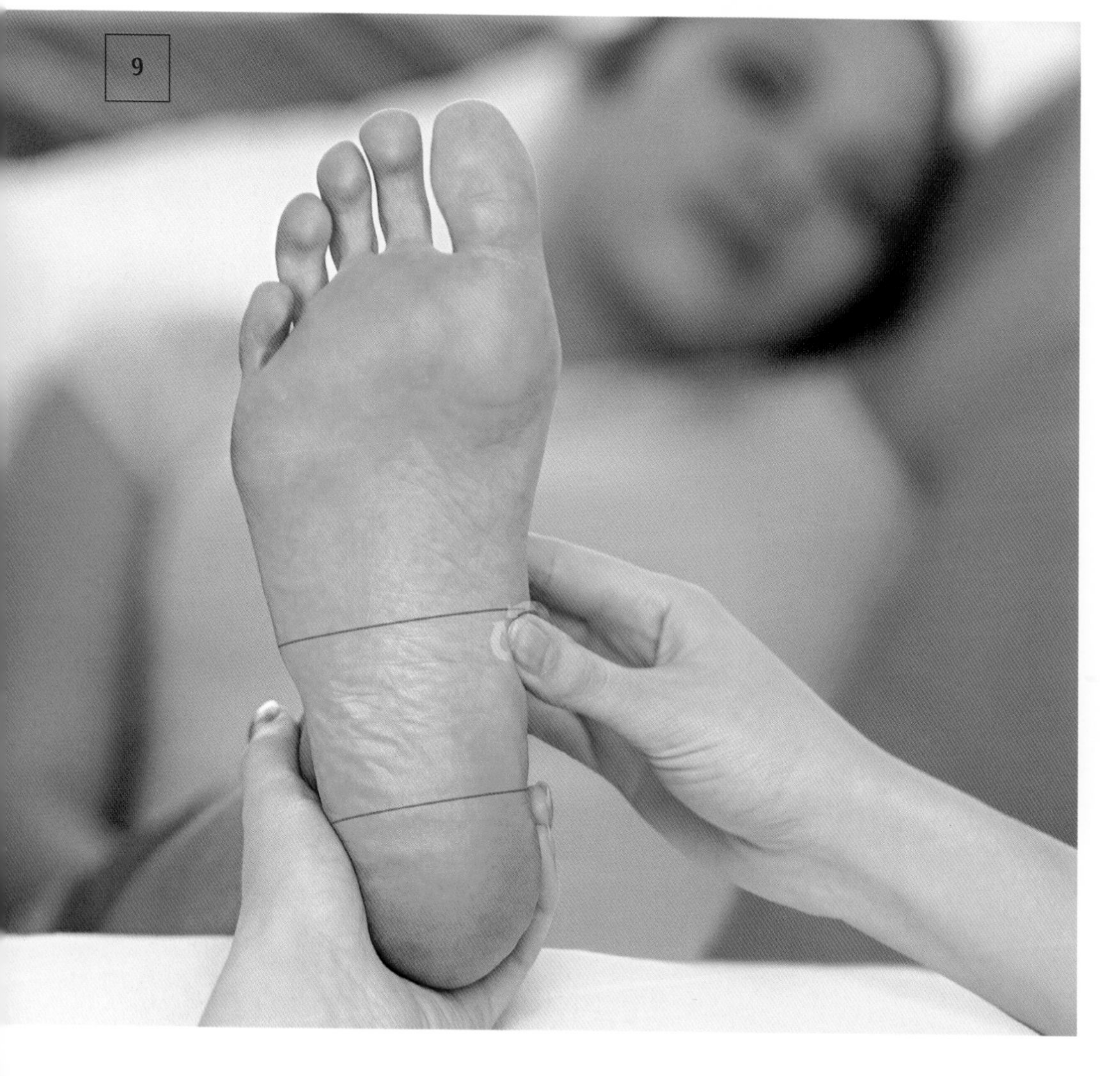

Simple exercises for your lower back

Regular exercise helps to keep your lower back mobile. If you do have lower back pain, the cat pose, followed by the child pose to rest your spine, can be very helpful.

Cat pose

Get down on your hands and knees. Make sure that your hands are positioned directly beneath your shoulders, and your knees are beneath your hips. Keep your back flat and look down at the floor.

Breathe in and curve your spine toward the ceiling, letting your head dip toward the floor (1). Hold for a few breaths. As you breathe out, gently drop your back down into an arch (2). Bring your head up and look straight ahead.

Child pose

Sit back on your heels and rest your forehead on the floor. Stretch your arms out in front of you and rest like this, breathing quietly, for about three minutes (3).

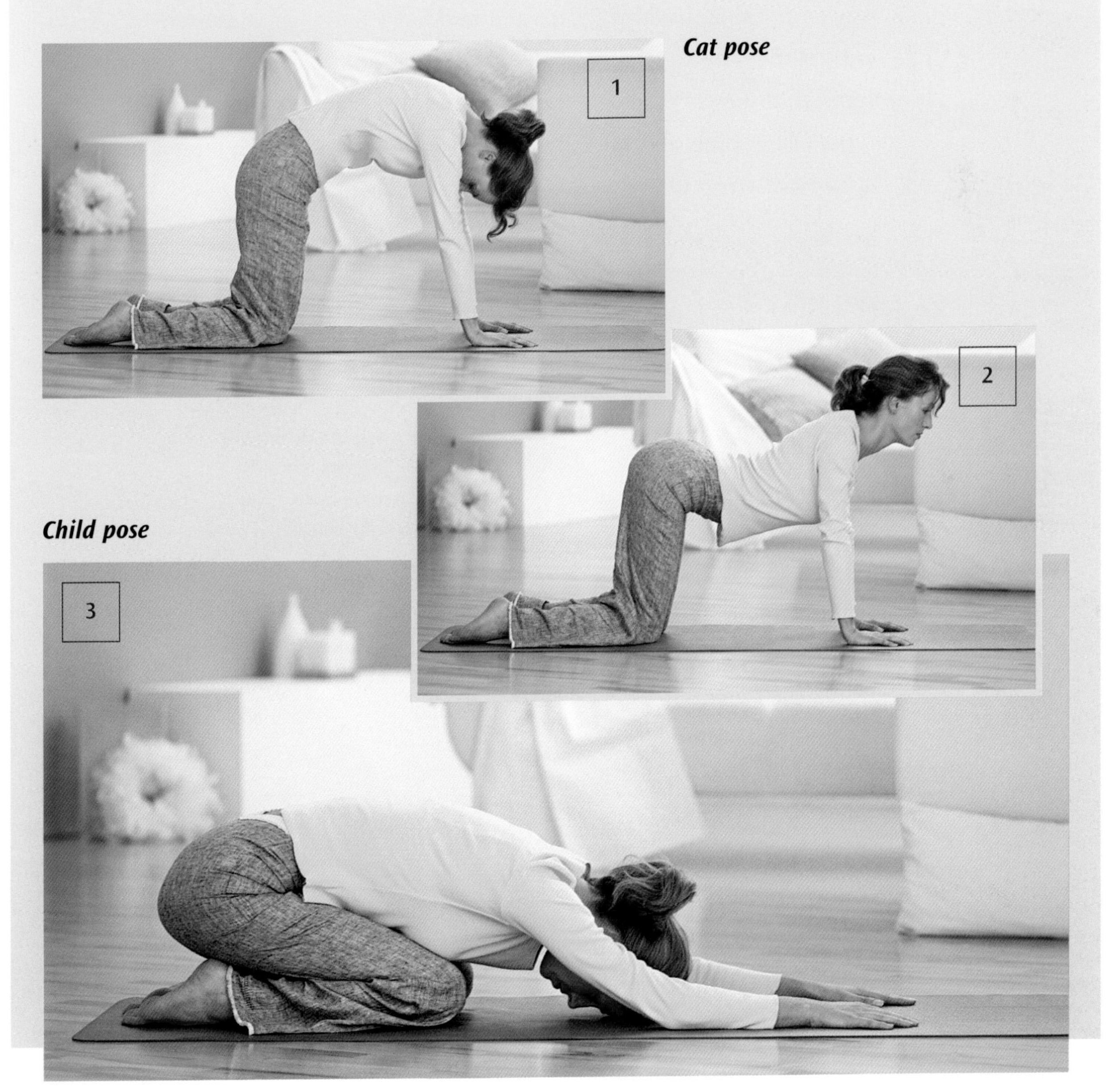

Cat pose

Child pose

TREATING THE KNEE & ELBOW

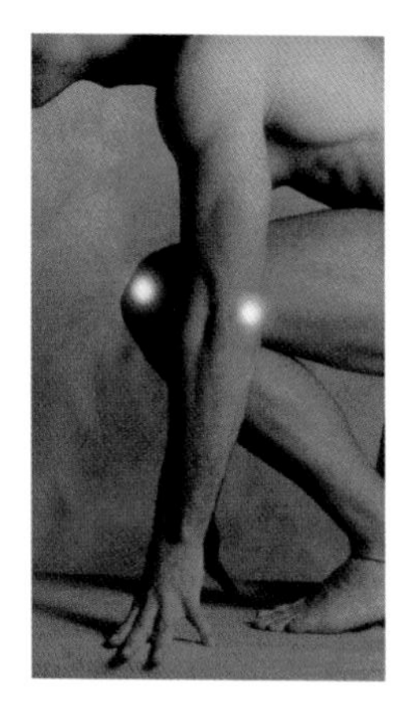

Hinge joints
The knee and the elbow are both hinge joints—they operate to bend or extend the legs and arms. The knee is a more complex joint than the elbow since it can also rotate slightly.

The knee is one of the largest joints in the body. It needs to be both stable to support the body's weight, and very flexible to allow movements such as walking, crouching, running, jumping, and turning. The knee is the only joint in the body that's capable of moving forward and backward, although in practice this is prevented by the kneecap, or patella, which fits into the knee hinge almost like a wedge. If the kneecap is broken, the lower leg is able to come forward.

The elbow joints allow the arms to bend and straighten, but are not subjected to as much pressure and wear and tear as the knees.

Because the knees have to do so much, they are very susceptible to damage. There are two main kinds of knee problems—mechanical, caused by accident and injury—and inflammatory—caused by conditions such as bursitis and arthritis. Reflexology can help ease knee pain, whatever the reason.

Knee injuries

Knee injuries from playing sports are common. The knee cartilage that cushions the bones of the knee can become torn or damaged; the joint can be dislocated by too much strain; and ligaments and muscles can be torn. After any of these injuries, rest your knee as much as you can and apply ice packs (see page 82) several times a day.

Chondromalacia

Chondromalacia is a condition that affects the cartilage at the back of the kneecap and is linked to overuse. It's common in runners, skiers, cyclists, and people who play ball games, and happens most often to teenagers and young adults. Symptoms of chondromalacia include pain under or around the kneecap that may be made worse by walking downstairs or downhill, as well as stiffness and cracking noises when the knee is moved. Usually only one knee is affected, and the condition generally gets better in a few months. Severe cases sometimes need surgery. Gentle exercise to strengthen the muscles will help and ice packs help to soothe the pain and inflammation.

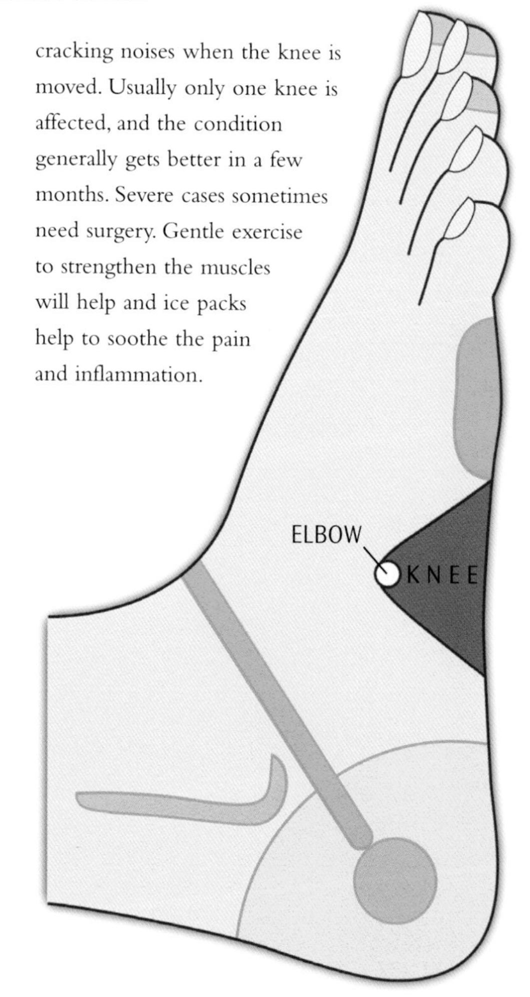

Areas on the foot
The knee and elbow share the same triangular-shaped reflex point on the side of the foot.

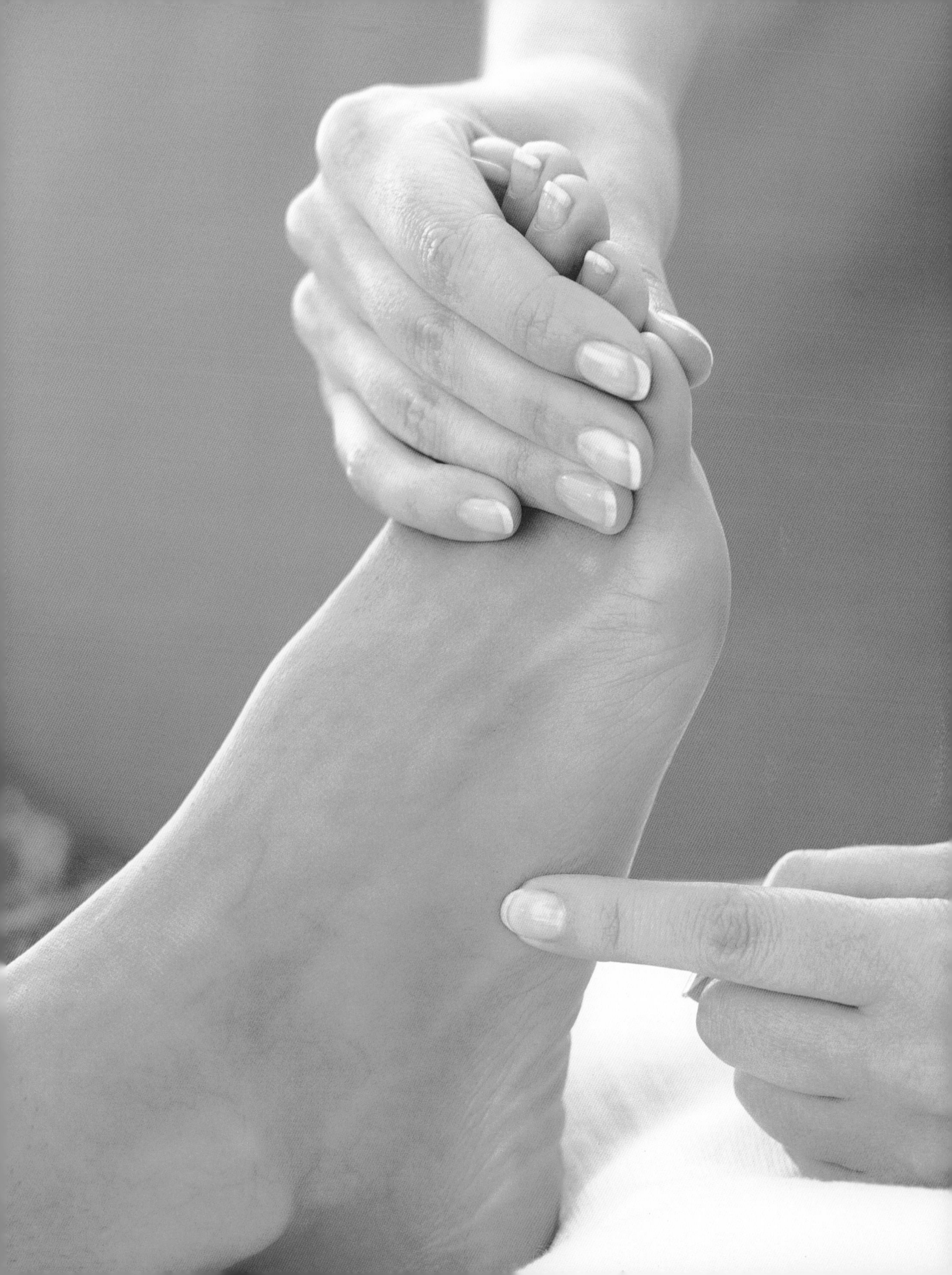

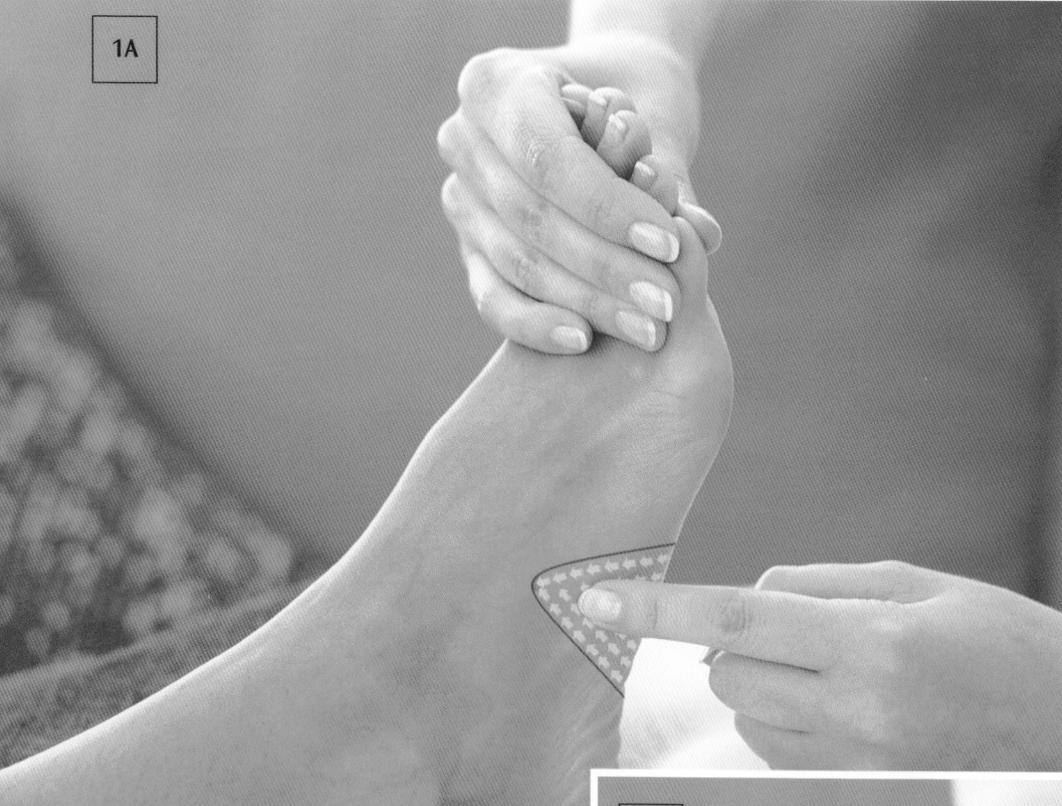

Knee and elbow

Support the right foot with your right hand. Using your left index finger, gently creep across the whole of the triangular knee and elbow reflex area on the outside of the foot (1A, 1B). The knee reflex is at the top of the triangle. The elbow reflex lies within the triangular area (see page 102). Switch hands to treat the left foot.

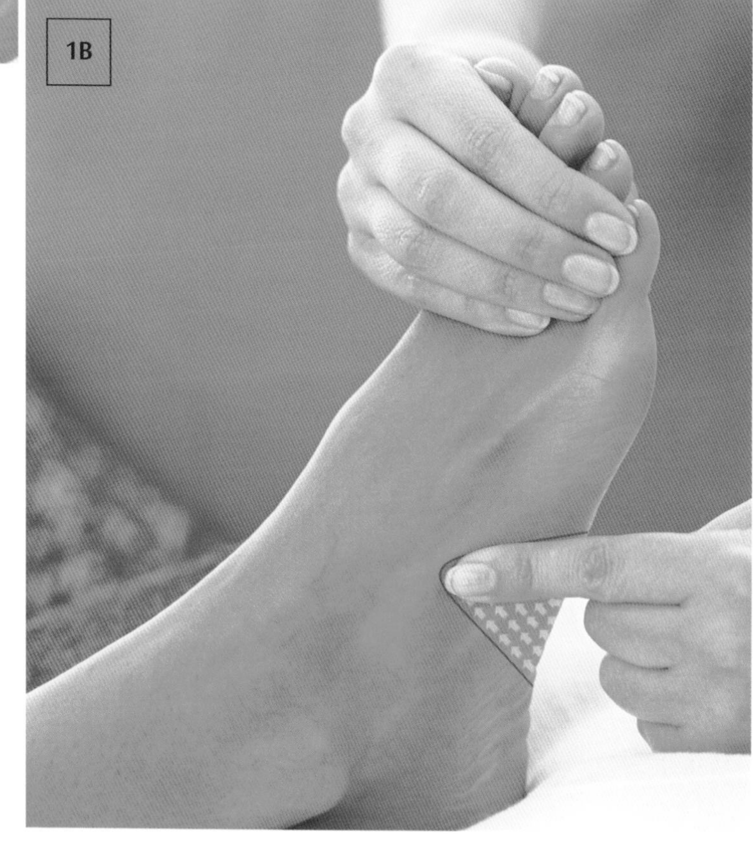

Bursitis

Bursae are small fluid-filled sacs in the knee that help it move smoothly. Prolonged or repeated stress on the knee, such as kneeling for a long time, can cause a condition called bursitis. (In the days when many women spent long hours on their hands and knees scrubbing floors, bursitis was known as housemaid's knee.)

In bursitis, the bursae become inflamed, and sometimes swollen, restricting the movement of the joint and causing pain. People suffering from conditions such as gout or rheumatoid arthritis tend to be at greater risk for bursitis. Bursitis can also affect the elbow joint.

Osteoarthritis

Osteoarthritis in the knee joints is all too common. Sufferers may have pain, swelling, and find they're not able to move their knees as well as they should. Arthritic knees may be particularly stiff in the morning and gradually ease with movement. Sometimes the joint locks and clicks when the knee is bent and straightened.

Arthritis in the knee may be caused by excess stress on the joint from repeated injury or extra weight. Osteoarthritis most often affects older and middle-aged people. A young person who develops osteoarthritis may have an inherited form of the disease or may have had repeated injuries to the knees.

Keep your knees healthy

Taking good care of your knees will help you avoid problems and injuries. Here are some suggestions.

Always warm up with a few stretches before playing sports or working out in the gym. Cool down afterward, too, with some more stretches after exercising and you're less likely to strain or injure your muscles.

Keep your leg muscles strong by exercising. The weaker your muscles are, the harder your knees have to work, and that puts them under stress and makes them more vulnerable to injury.

Check your posture. Walking and standing badly puts strain on your knees.

The health of your knees is yet another reason to keep your weight down. The heavier you are, the bigger the load for your knees to carry, and they are likely to suffer.

Elbow pain

A common elbow problem is tennis elbow. This happens when the tendon in the elbow gets damaged and inflamed and can be caused by any excessive or repetitive strain on the joint, not just playing tennis.

In tennis elbow the tendon on the outside of the elbow is damaged. In golfer's elbow it is the tendon on the inside of the elbow. In both cases it will help to rest the elbow and treat with ice packs as well as reflexology.

A simple treatment for your knees and elbows

A castor oil pack is a good, old-fashioned remedy for painful arthritic knees and elbows. The castor oil draws out impurities from the joint and brings great relief from pain.

You can buy special castor oil packs, but it's easy to make one for yourself.

Put three tablespoons of castor oil into a small basin. Place the basin over a pan of boiling water and heat it gently. Take a thick wad of cotton, soak it in the warm oil, and place this over the painful joint. Cover the area with plastic wrap to keep the pad in place and help retain the warmth of the oil. Make sure you cover the whole castor oil pad with plastic wrap since the oil will stain anything it touches.

Wrap a towel around the whole area and leave on overnight. Alternatively, you can place a heating pad over the castor oil pack and leave on for a couple of hours.

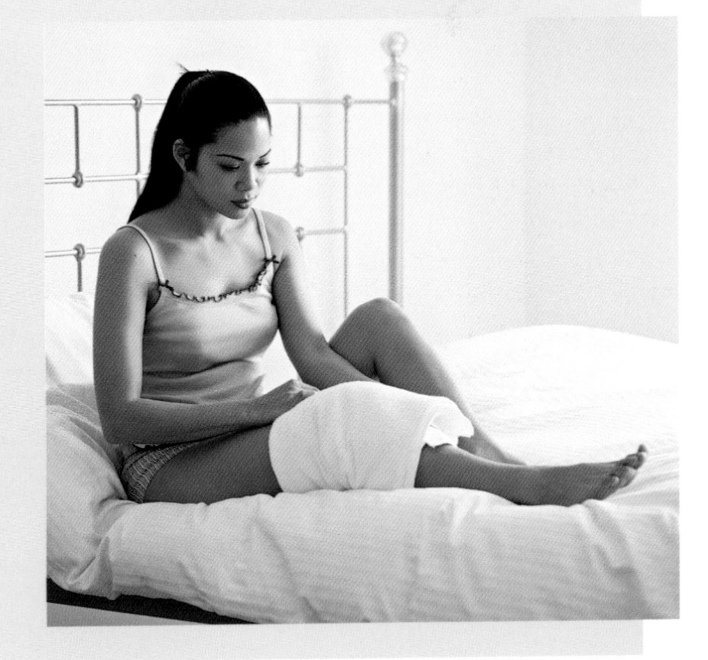

TREATING CHRONIC & BACK CONDITIONS

Nearly everyone has back pain at some time in their lives. Chronic back pain becomes more likely as you get older and bone strength and muscle tone diminish, so it's vital to keep your back as healthy as possible.

A chronic back condition is one that lasts some time—say, more than three months or so. It may be the result of a disease that affects the health of the bones, such as osteoporosis or osteomalacia, or a condition such as ankylosing spondylitis. Problems with the spine, such as "slipped discs" can develop over a period of time and cause great pain.

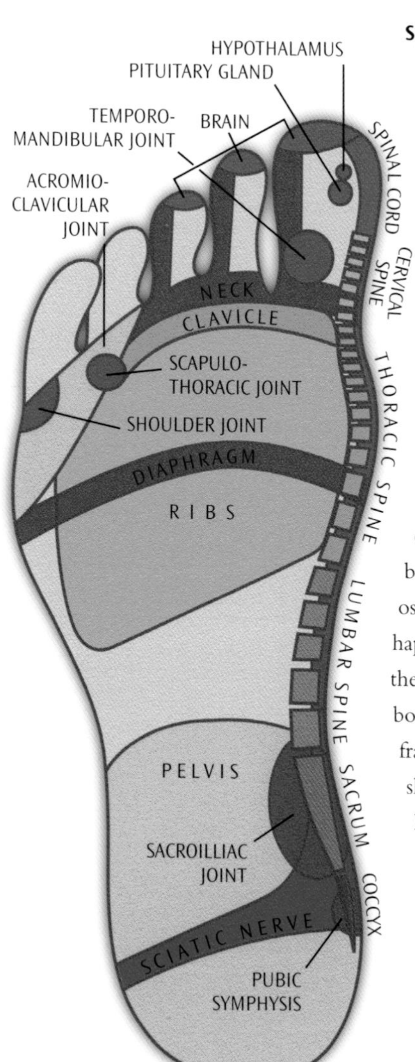

Areas on the foot
Work on these reflex points for the spine and hips to ease chronic back pain.

The following conditions are some of the most common causes of chronic back pain.

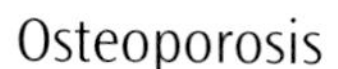

Osteoporosis

As you get older, your bones get thinner and lighter as the body's ability to replace bone declines. Healthy bones are dense and contain plenty of calcium and other minerals. Bones affected by osteoporosis lack minerals and become brittle and porous—osteoporosis means porous bones. This happens to everyone to some degree as they get older, but in some people the bones get so fragile that they break and fracture very easily. The whole skeleton may be affected, but bone loss is usually greatest in the spine, hips, and ribs. Since the spine and hips bear a great deal of weight, they are susceptible to pain, deformity, and fracture.

Osteoporosis itself does not cause back pain. But it can result in pain if the vertebrae become so weak that they can no longer withstand normal stresses applied to them, or the sufferer has an accident, such as a fall.

Women are four times more likely than men to develop osteoporosis and the condition is particularly common in post-menopausal white women. One symptom is a considerable reduction in height.

Is osteoporosis preventable?

It certainly is. While there has been a great push to encourage people to take calcium in an effort to halt bone loss, osteoporosis is much more than a lack of dietary calcium. It is a complex condition involving hormonal, lifestyle, nutritional, and environmental factors. People who have a good calcium-rich diet and do regular weight-bearing exercise earlier in life are far less likely to suffer osteoporosis later.

A common cause of calcium loss in people in the Western world today is the huge intake of carbonated drinks, such as colas. Many of these

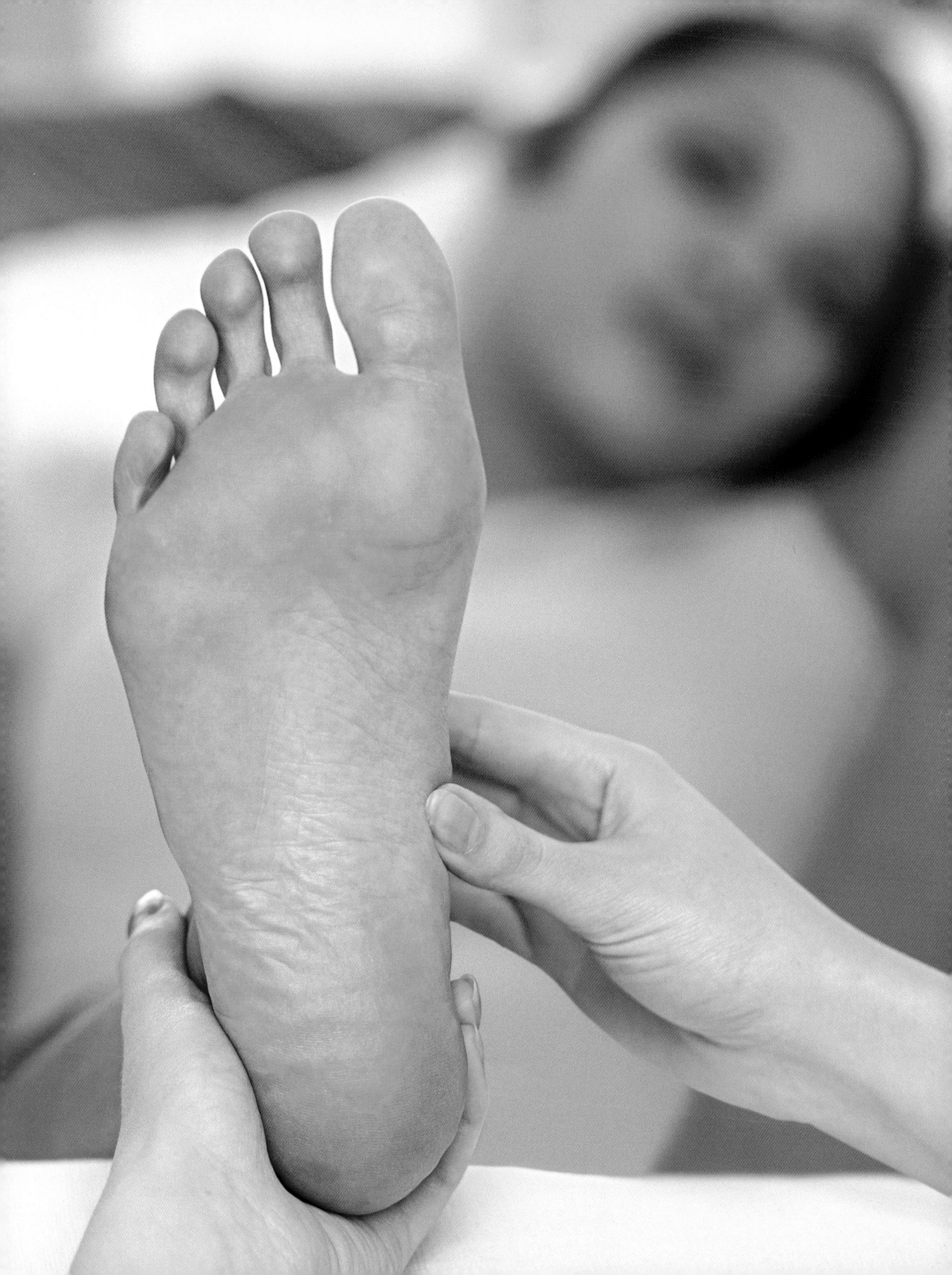

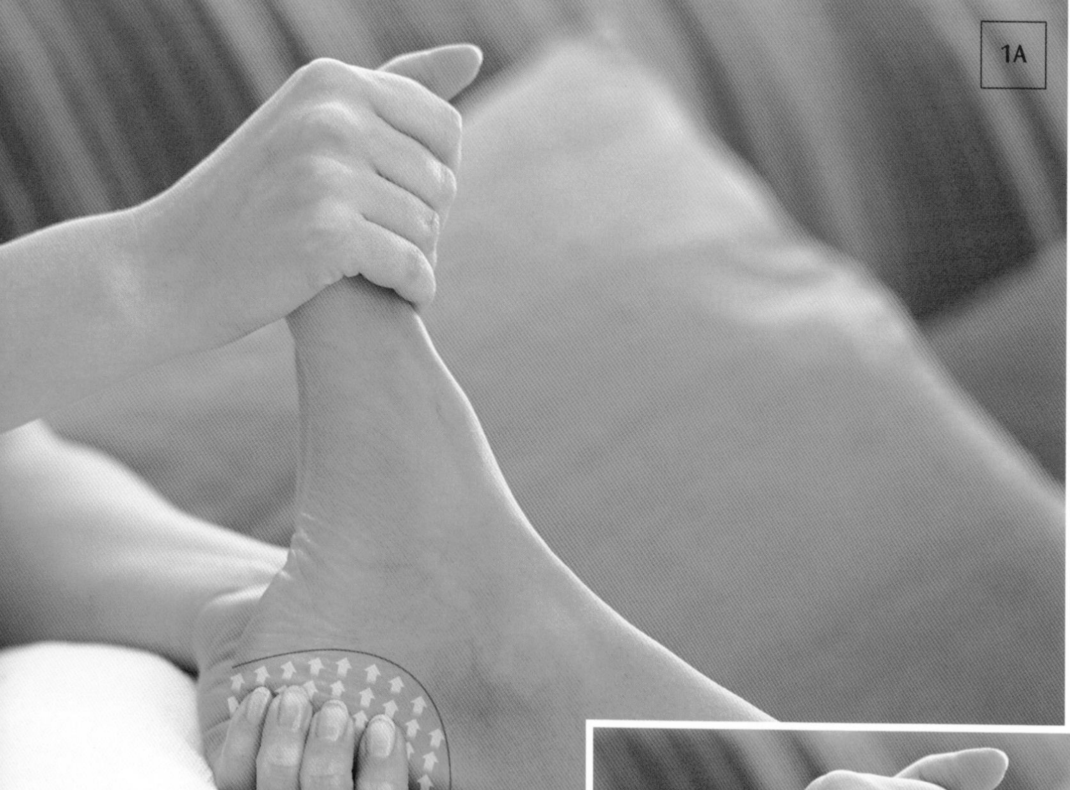

Coccyx

Spine work generally starts with the coccyx. Hold the top of the right foot with your right hand. Place all four fingers of the left hand on the coccyx area and make small creeping movements up the inside of the heel (1A, 1B). Switch hands to treat the left foot.

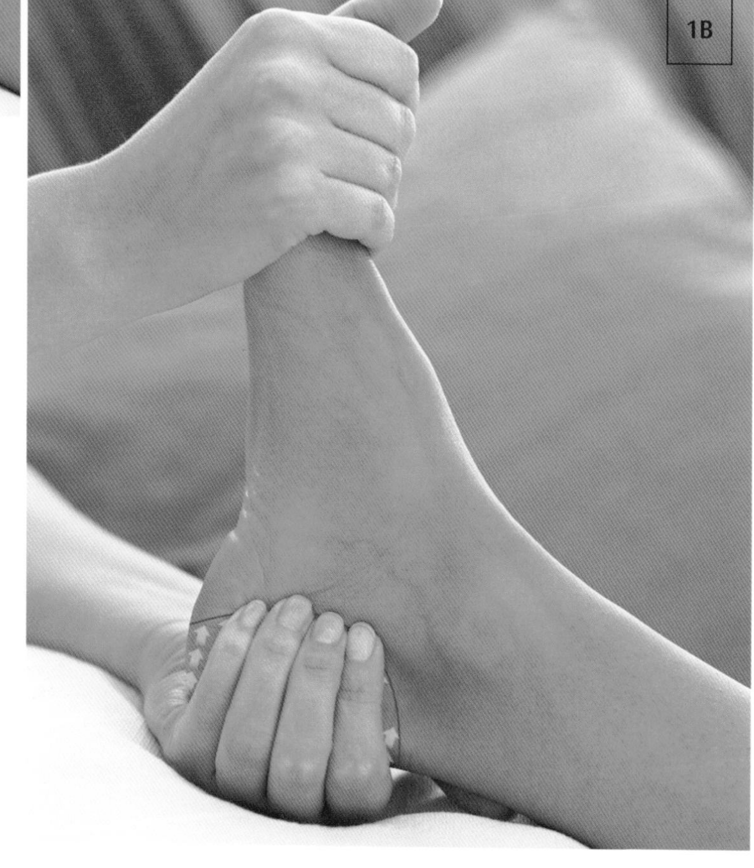

drinks contain phosphoric acid, which leaches calcium out of bone and affects bone mass. If you want healthy bones, avoid carbonated drinks.

Steroids are another cause of bone loss and it is worrisome to think that as many as one in five of young children today is using an inhaler containing steroid medications to control asthma. No wonder doctors are seeing bone loss in children.

It is essential to build bone mass and protect our bones when young and not leave it until symptoms start appearing. Prevention is always better than cure. If you suffer from osteoporosis, back massage, which increases the blood supply to the muscles in the spine, can help to relieve discomfort.

Osteomalacia

Osteomalacia is also known as "soft bone."
It is caused by a lack of vitamin D, either because of insufficient intake or the inability to absorb the

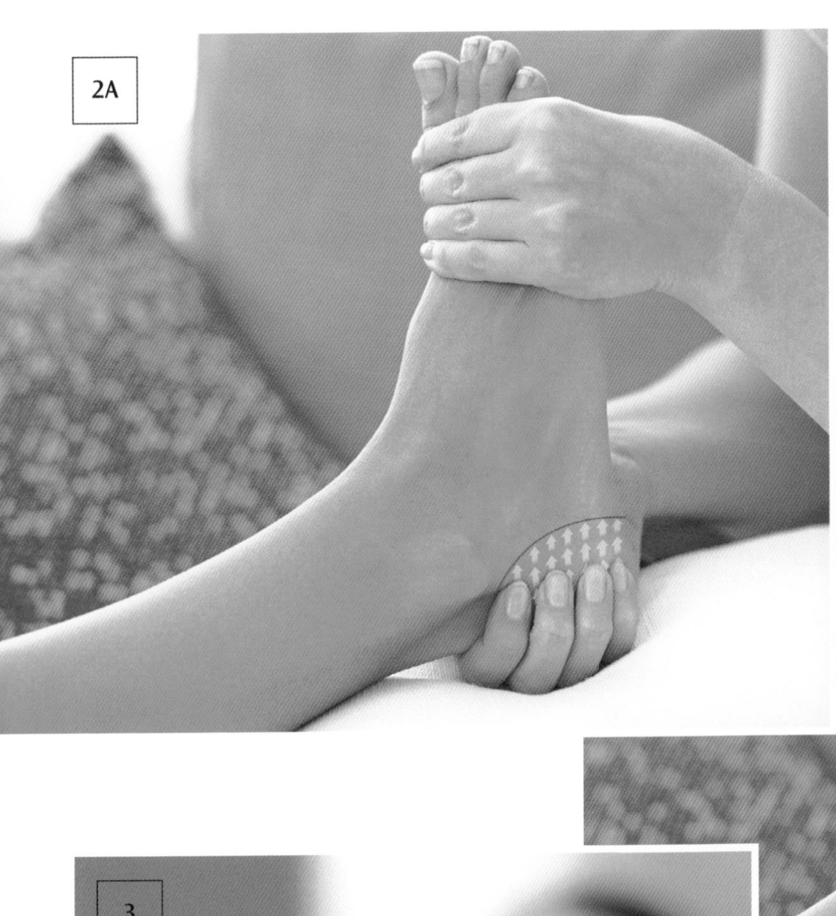

Hip and pelvis (lateral)

To work the hip and pelvis, support the top of the right foot with your left hand. Using the four fingers of your right hand, creep up the lateral side of the heel (2A, 2B). Switch hands to treat the left foot.

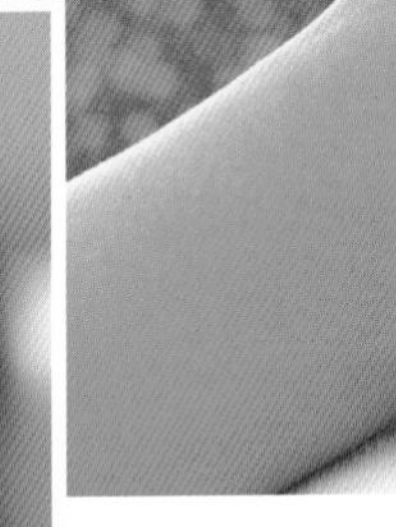

Hip and pelvis (plantar)

Supporting the right foot in the palm of the right hand, work across the base of the heel (3). These reflex points represent the back of the pelvis. Switch hands to treat the left foot.

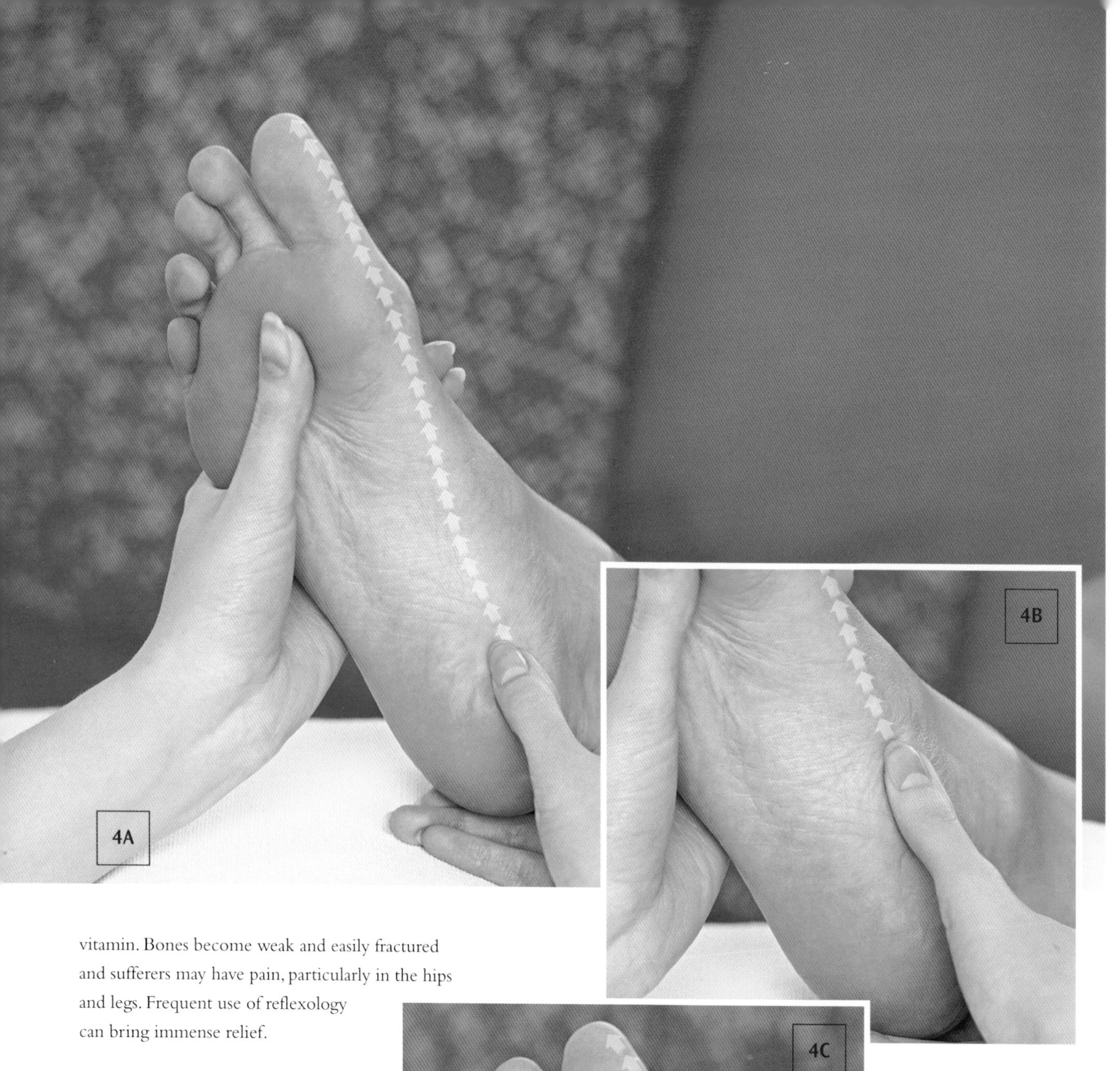

vitamin. Bones become weak and easily fractured and sufferers may have pain, particularly in the hips and legs. Frequent use of reflexology can bring immense relief.

Ankylosing spondylitis

Ankylosing spondylitis is a relatively rare condition that affects the spine as well as sacroiliac joints in the pelvis. The joints become inflamed and new bone starts to grow between the joints, which start to fuse together, making movement difficult. Multiple small stress fractures may develop and gravity tends to tip the body forward, so the patient may develop a forward posture. This condition typically affects young males. Sufferers are usually advised to take

Spine (up)

To treat back conditions, always work up the spine, then down. Working in both directions greatly enhances the treatment. The spine reflex points follow the line of the medial edge of the foot—they are not on the sole. Support the right foot with your left hand. Using your right thumb, creep up the line of reflex points, starting at the base of the spine (4A, 4B, 4C).

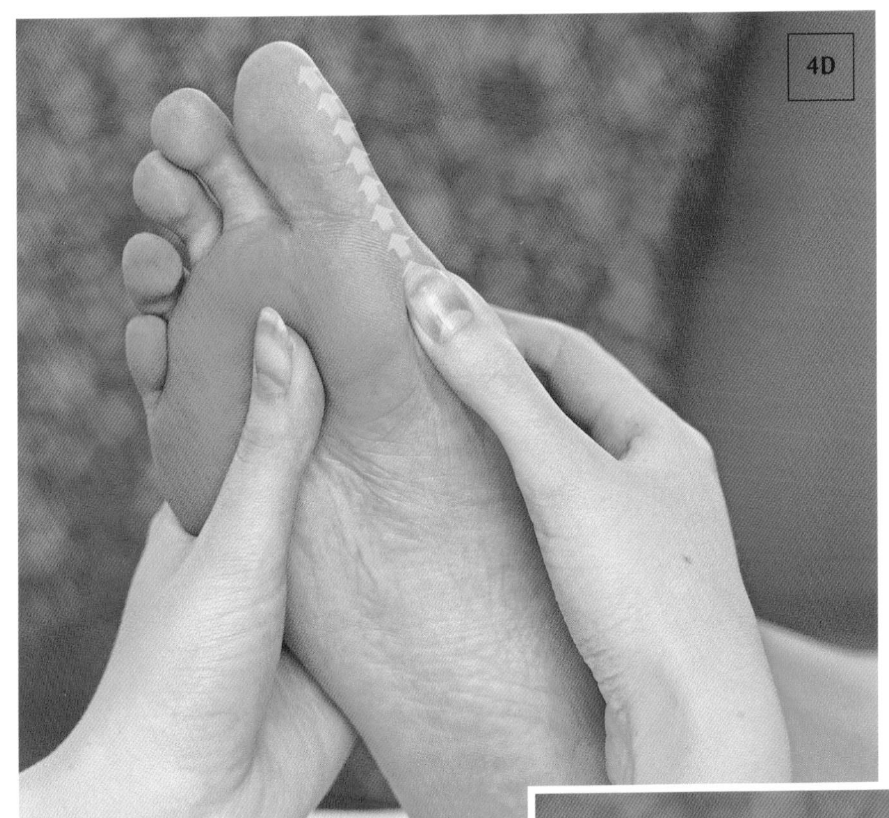

Spine (up)

Continue working up the spinal reflex points to the neck (4D, 4E). Switch hands to treat the left foot. This treatment helps all back conditions, including osteomalacia, spondylitis, and arthritis.

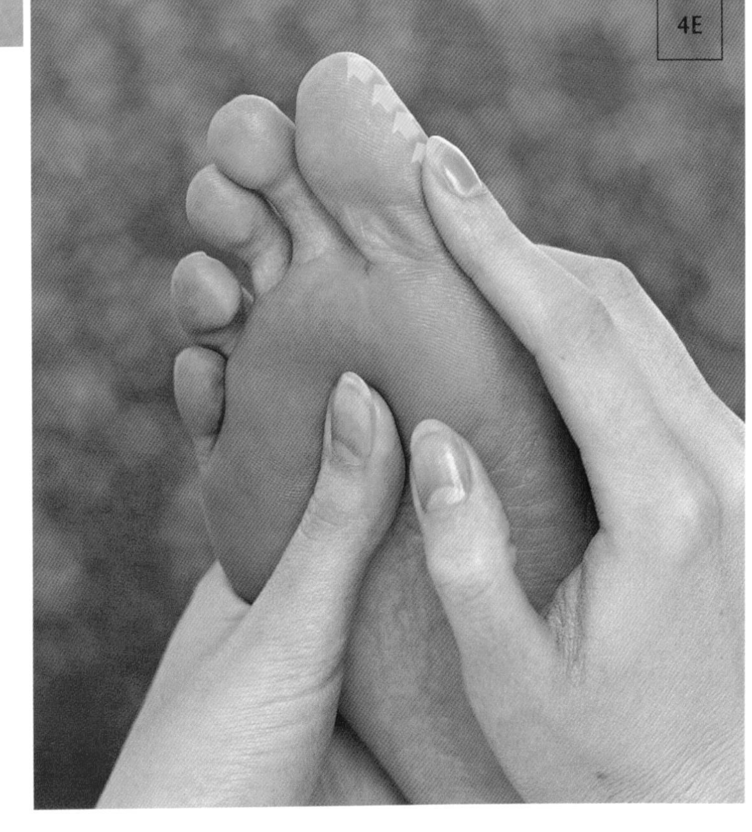

anti-inflammatory drugs and do special exercises to maintain some movement in the lumbar spine and hips.

Reflexology can certainly free the spine and most people with this condition have more flexibility and less pain after treatment. For the greatest benefit, people with ankylosing spondylitis should have regular reflexology treatment for an indefinite period.

Disc problems

The spinal discs are pads of cartilage that separate one bony vertebra from the next. In addition to keeping the vertebrae apart, the discs act as shock absorbers for the spine. Each disc is made up of a tough outer layer with a soft jelly-like core. As we get older the discs get thinner—one reason why people tend to shrink in height in old age.

Discs are under constant pressure, but they do not "slip." The condition referred to as slipped disc is

Spine (down)

After working up the spine, work down. Support the sole of the foot with the back of your nonworking hand. Use your thumb to creep down the medial edge of the foot, starting at the big toe (5A, 5B).

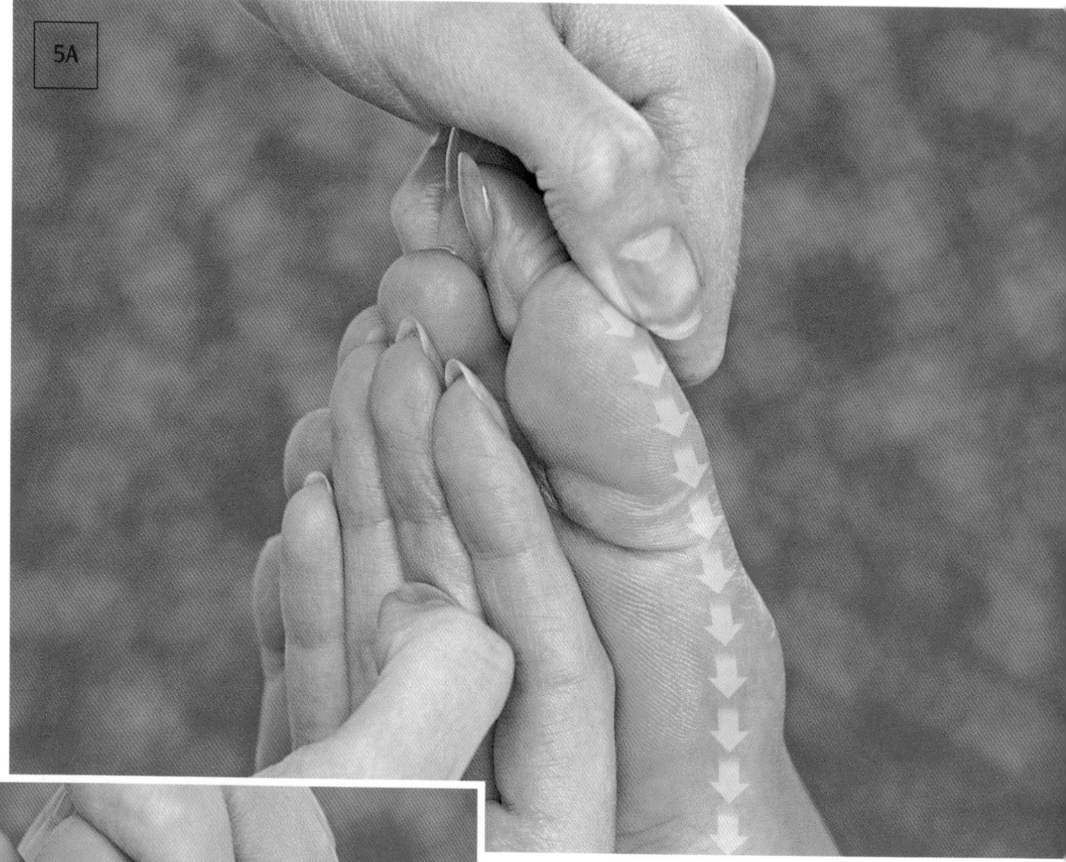

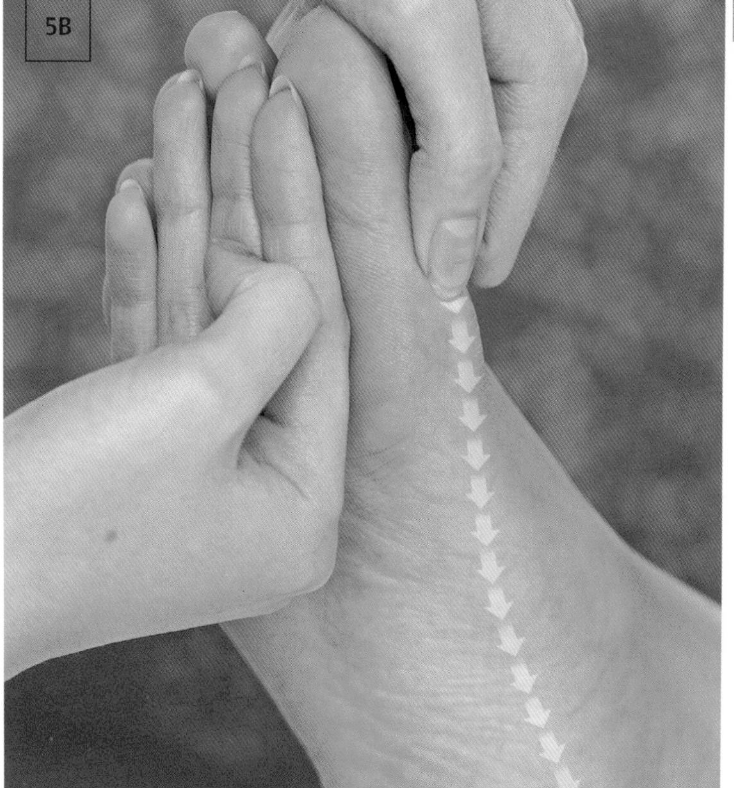

properly called a prolapsed or herniated disc. In this case, the soft core of the disc oozes out, distorting the disc. The surrounding area becomes inflamed and swollen and there may be pressure on a nerve—this is what causes pain.

Disc problems are most common in the lower back and symptoms may appear over some weeks or may start suddenly. They include severe pain in the back, or down the back of the leg, difficulty in moving, and muscle spasms. You'll be advised to rest in bed to give your disc a chance to recover. However, a weakness will remain in that area and you'll need to be sure to take extra care of your back in the future.

All pain and symptoms that affect the skeletal system will benefit by working out all the reflex areas described in this chapter.

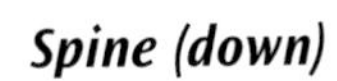

Spine (down)

Continue working down the medial edge of the foot with your thumb until you reach the heel (5C, 5D, 5E). Switch hands to treat the left foot.

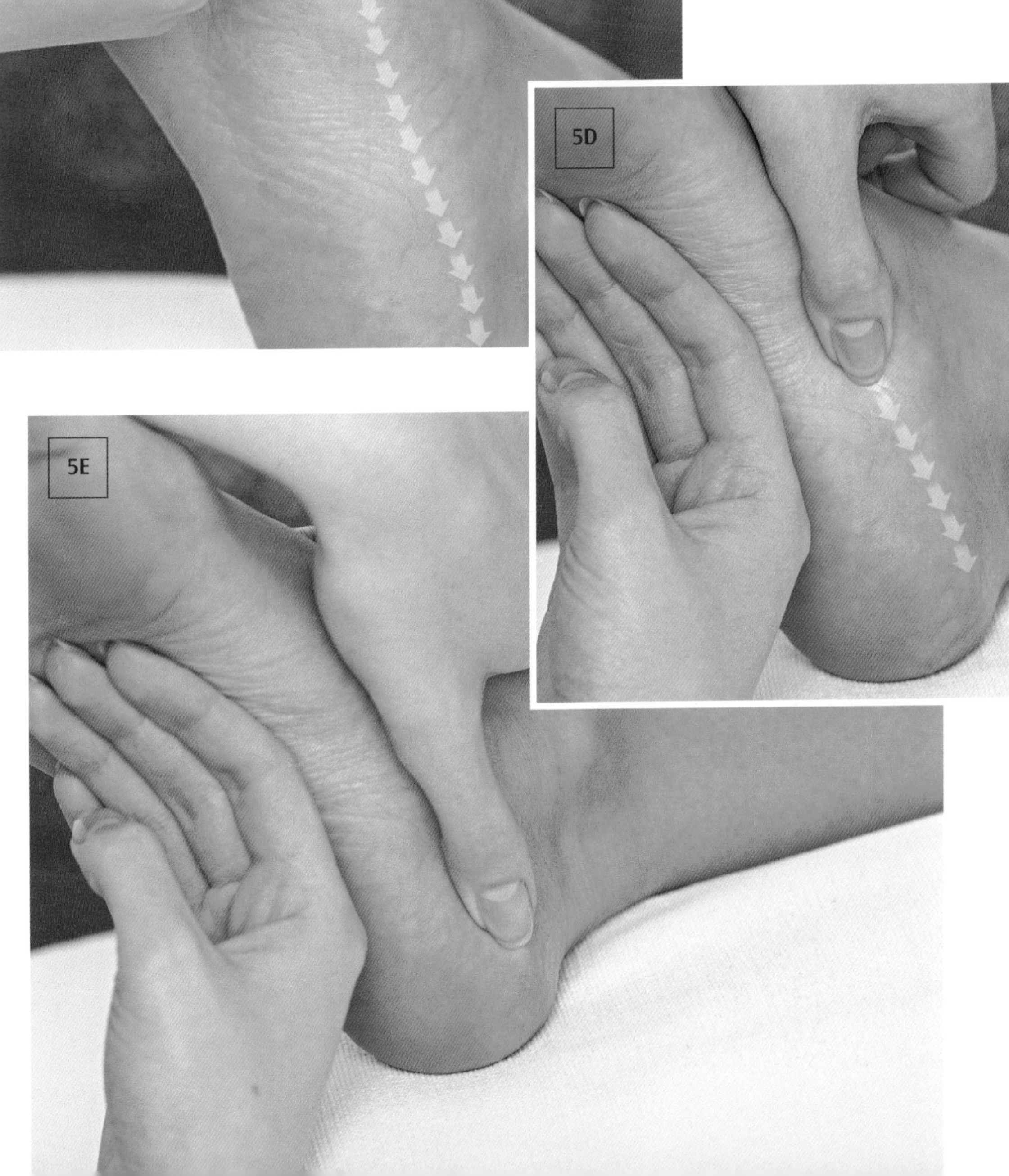

Chronic neck pain

To treat chronic neck pain, support the right foot with your left hand. Using the right thumb work down the outer edge of the first three toes (6A, 6B, 6C). Switch hands to treat the left foot.

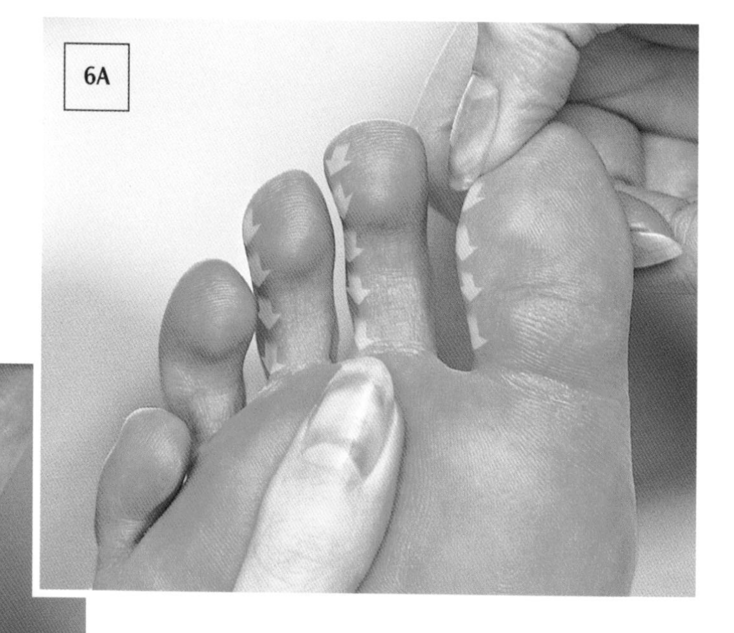

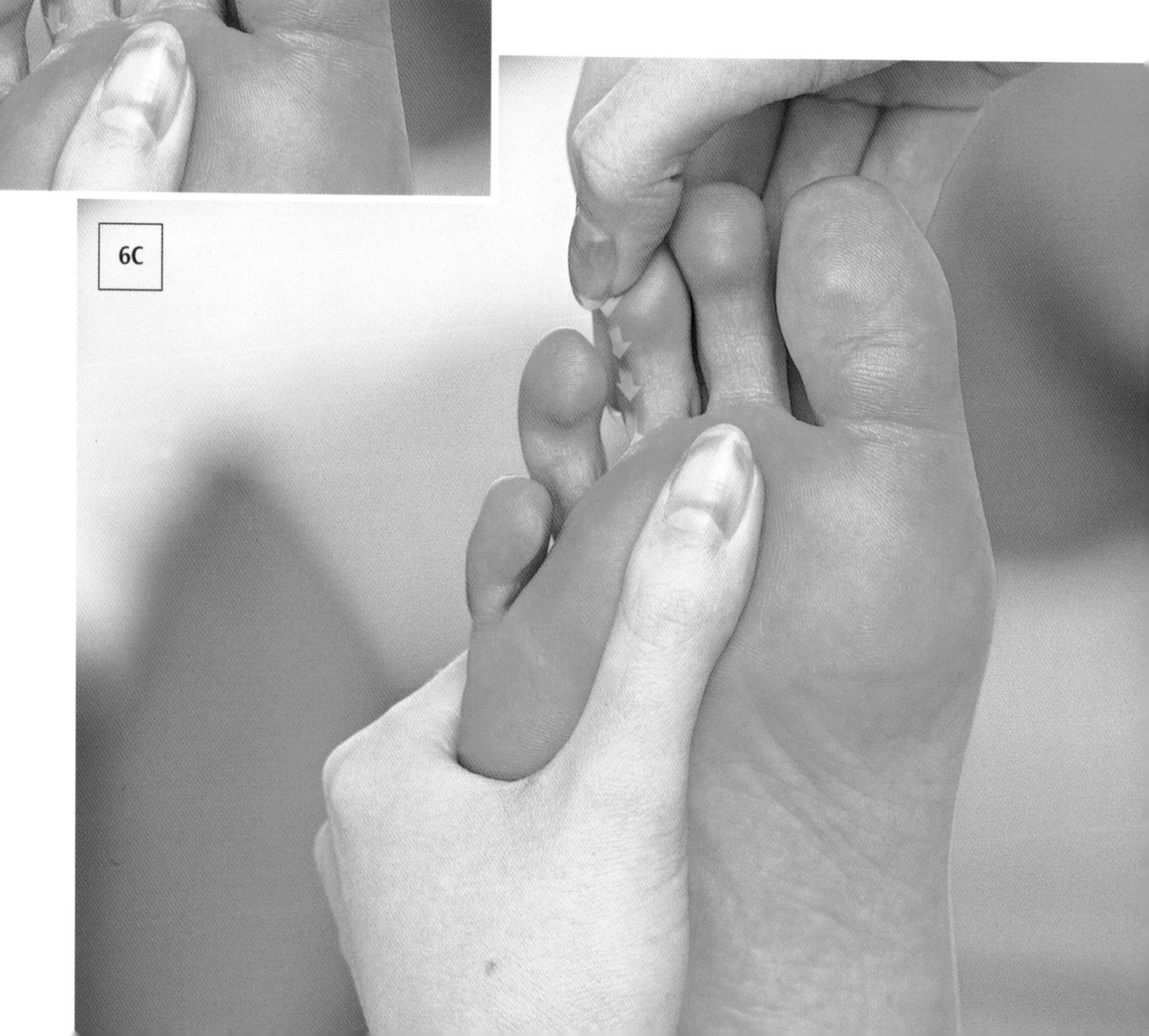

Neck pain (plantar)

To treat stiff necks, arthritis and whiplash injury, support the right foot with your left hand. Using your right thumb, work around the bases of the first three toes (7). Switch hands to treat the left foot.

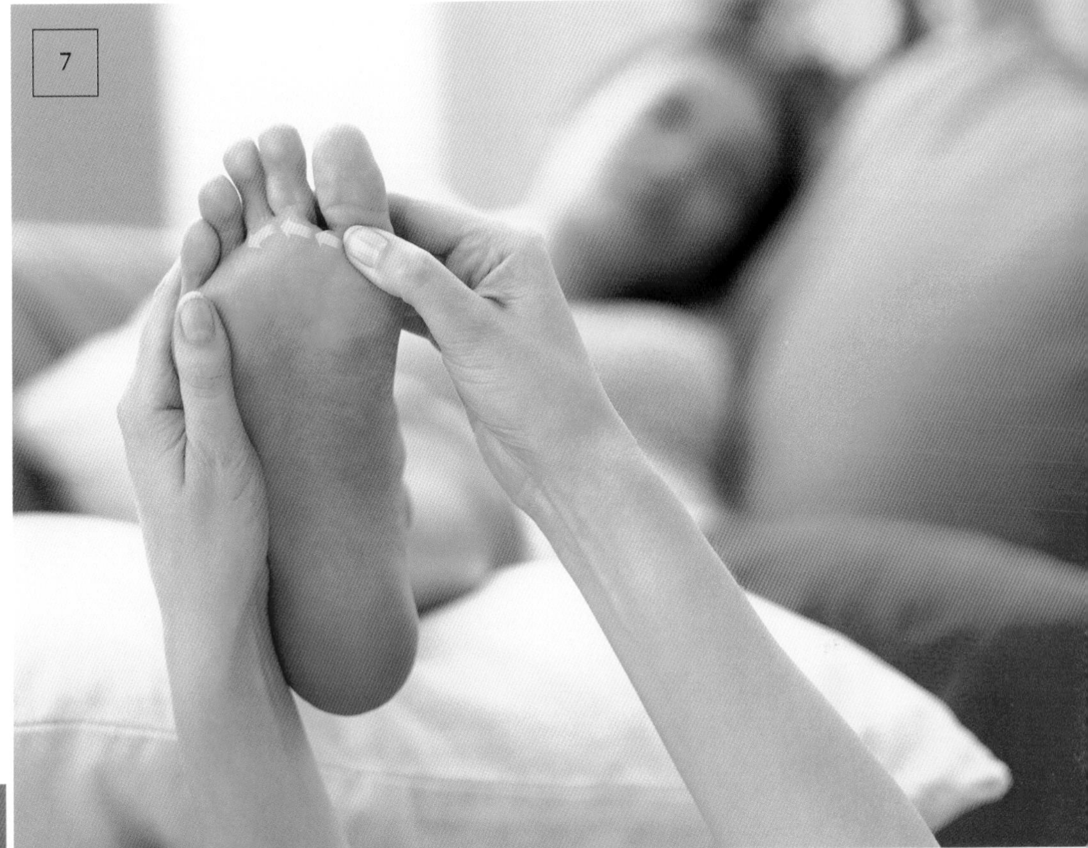

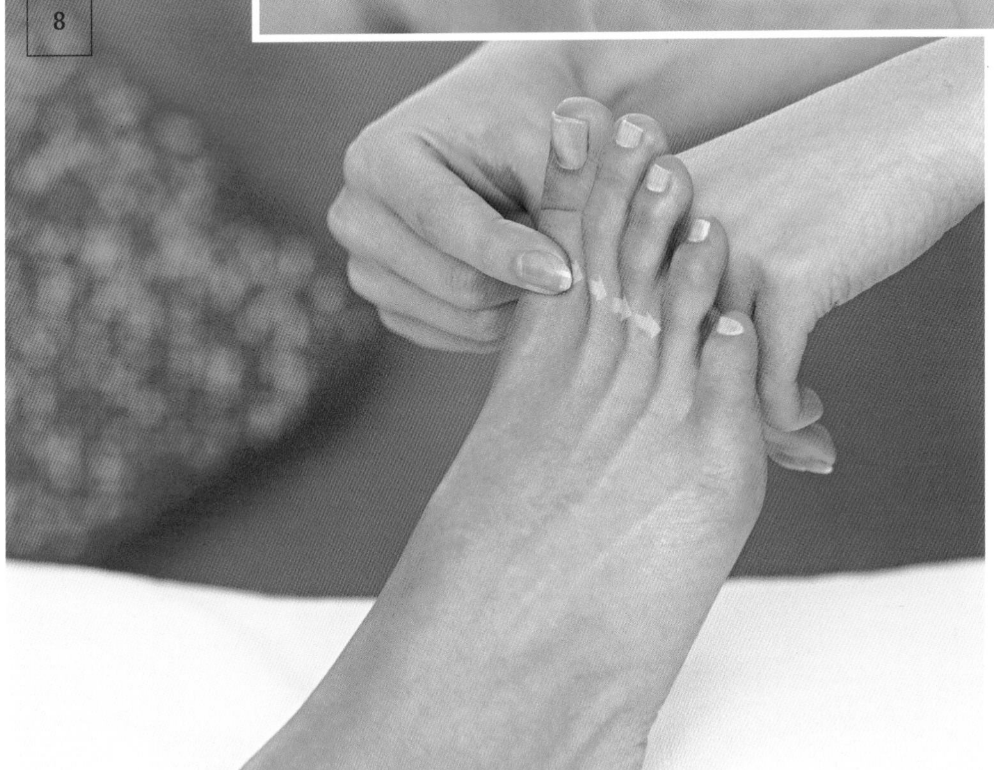

Neck pain (dorsal)

Make a fist with your left hand and press into the sole of the right foot. Using your right index finger, work on the bases of the first three toes (8). Switch hands to treat the left foot.

Shoulder (plantar)

For chronic shoulder pain, support the top of the right foot against your left hand. Using your right thumb, creep outward across the shoulder reflex area (9A). Change hands and support the foot with your right hand while creeping inward across the reflex area with your left thumb (9B). Switch hands to treat the left foot.

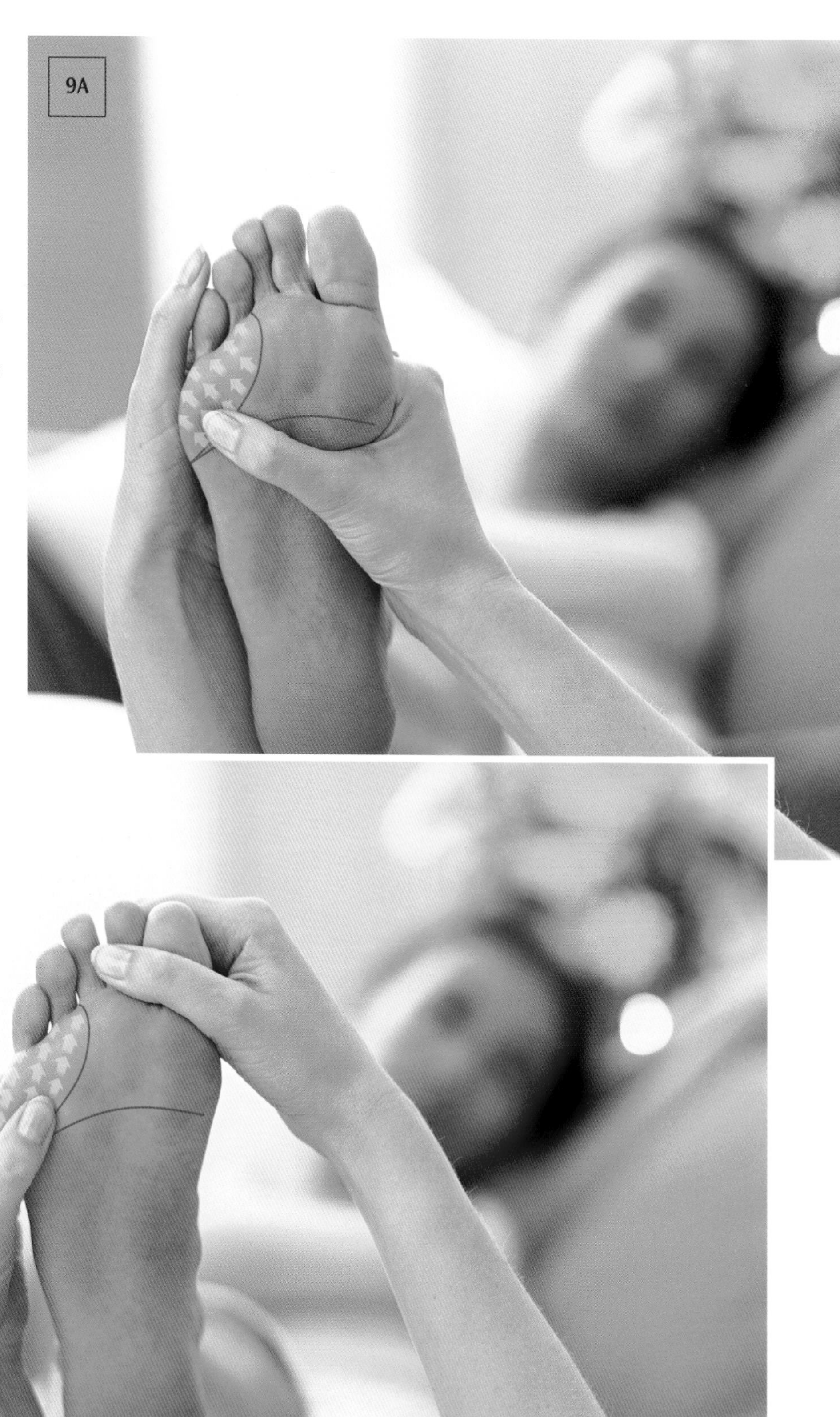

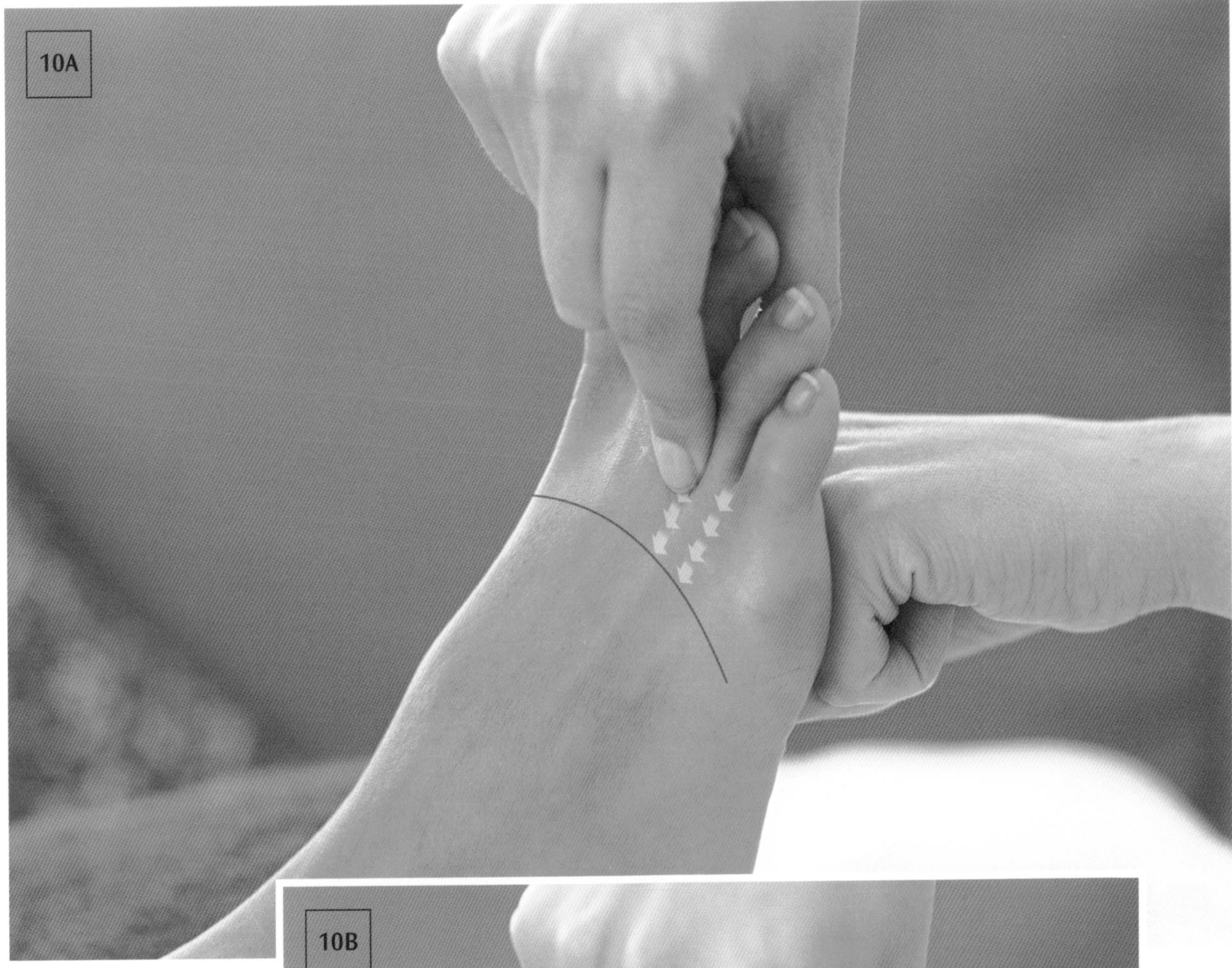

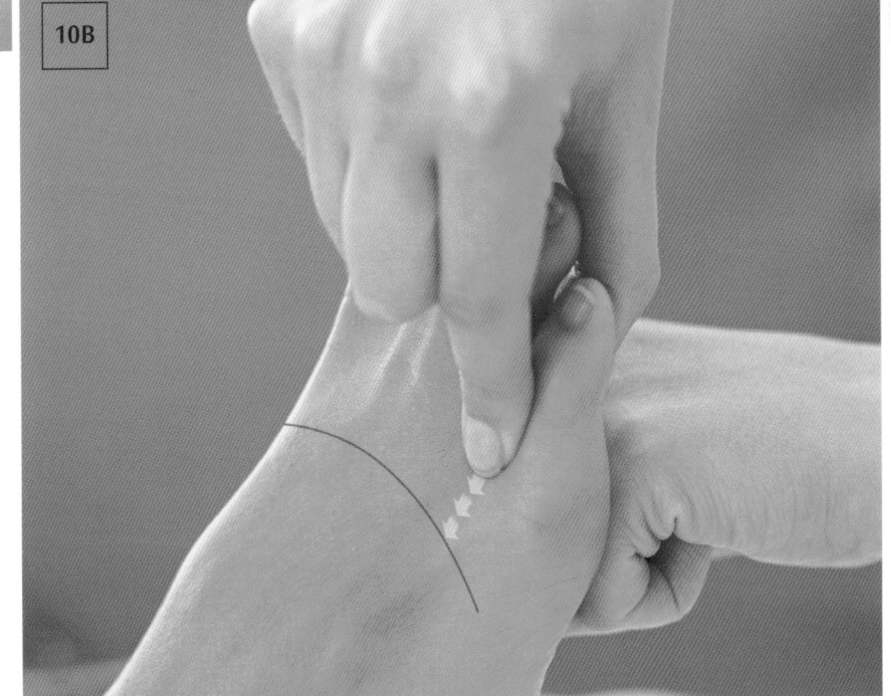

Shoulder (dorsal)

To treat the front of the shoulder joint, support the right foot against your left hand. Using your right index finger, work between the grooves of the fourth and fifth toes (10A, 10B). Switch hands to treat the left foot.

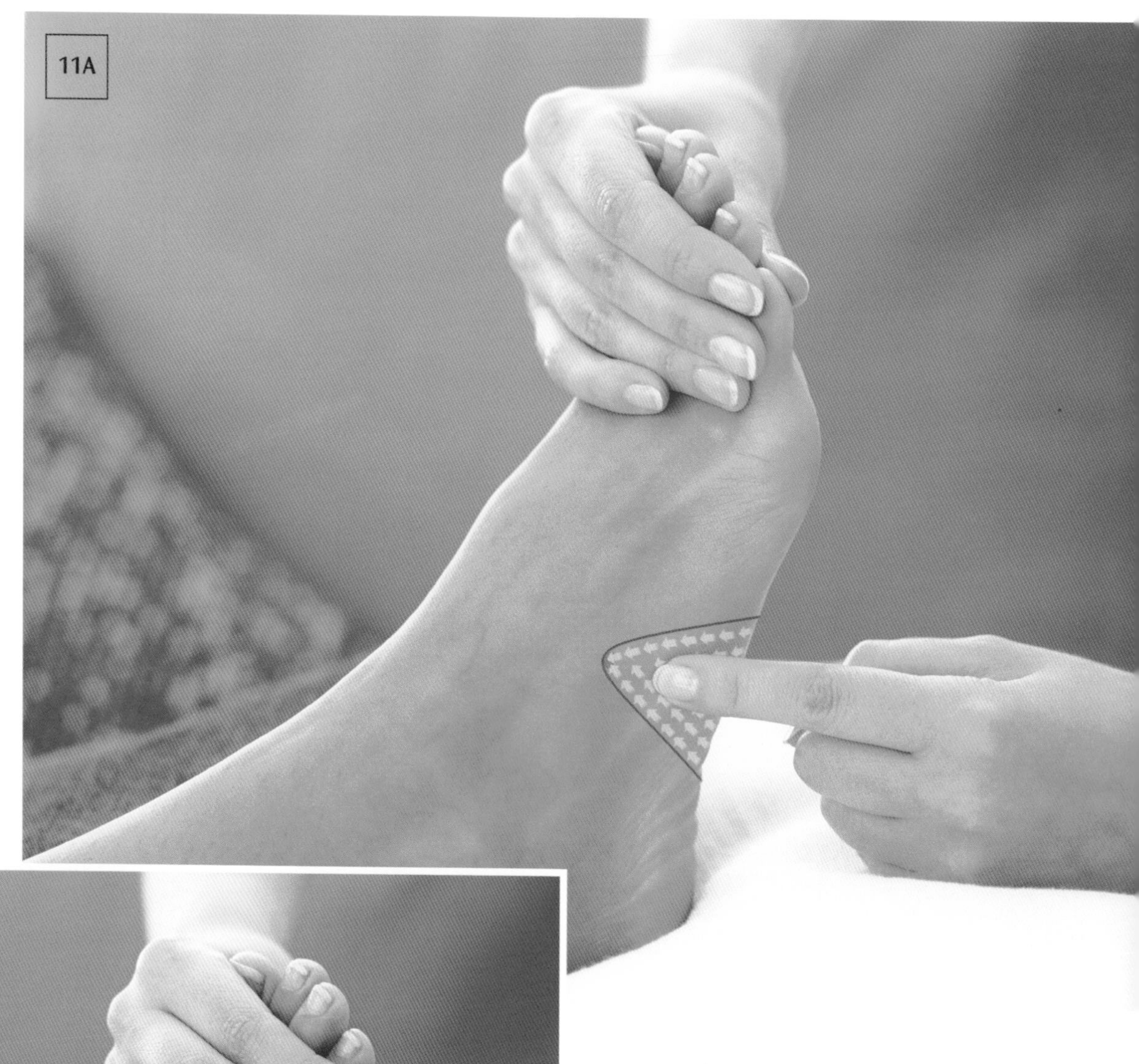

11B

Knee and elbow

For chronic knee and elbow pain, support the right foot with your right hand. Using your left index finger, creep across the triangular reflex area on the outside of the foot (11A). Continue working up to the top of the triangle that aligns with the bony protuberance you can feel on the side of the foot (11B). Switch hands to treat the left foot.

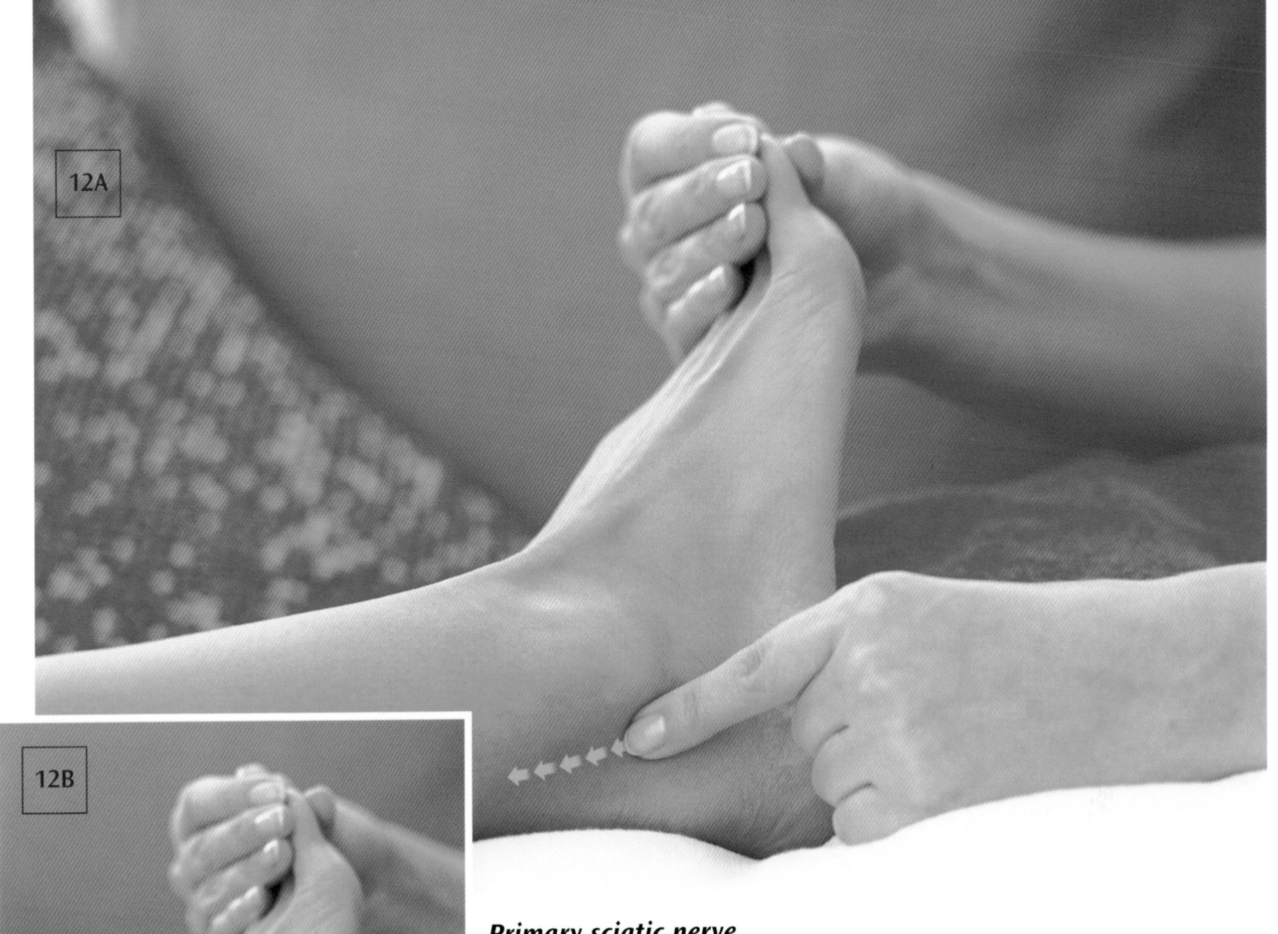

Primary sciatic nerve

To treat sciatic pain, hold the right foot with your right hand. Place your left index finger just behind the ankle bone. Creep up the leg for about 1½ inches (4 cm) (12A, 12B). Switch hands to treat the left foot.

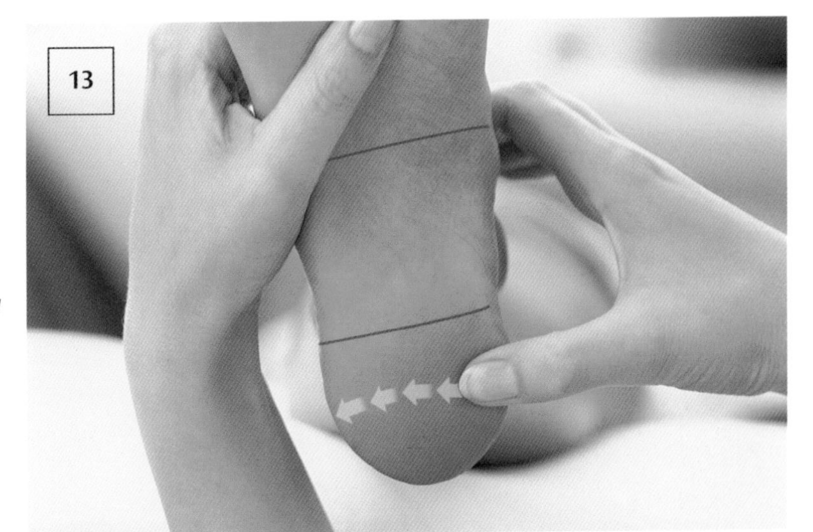

Secondary sciatic

The secondary sciatic reflex point lies across the heel, about halfway between the pelvic line (see page 18) and the bottom of the foot. To treat the sciatic nerve route, use your thumb to creep along this line two or three times. Work from the inside to the outside edge of the foot (13). Switch hands to treat the left foot.

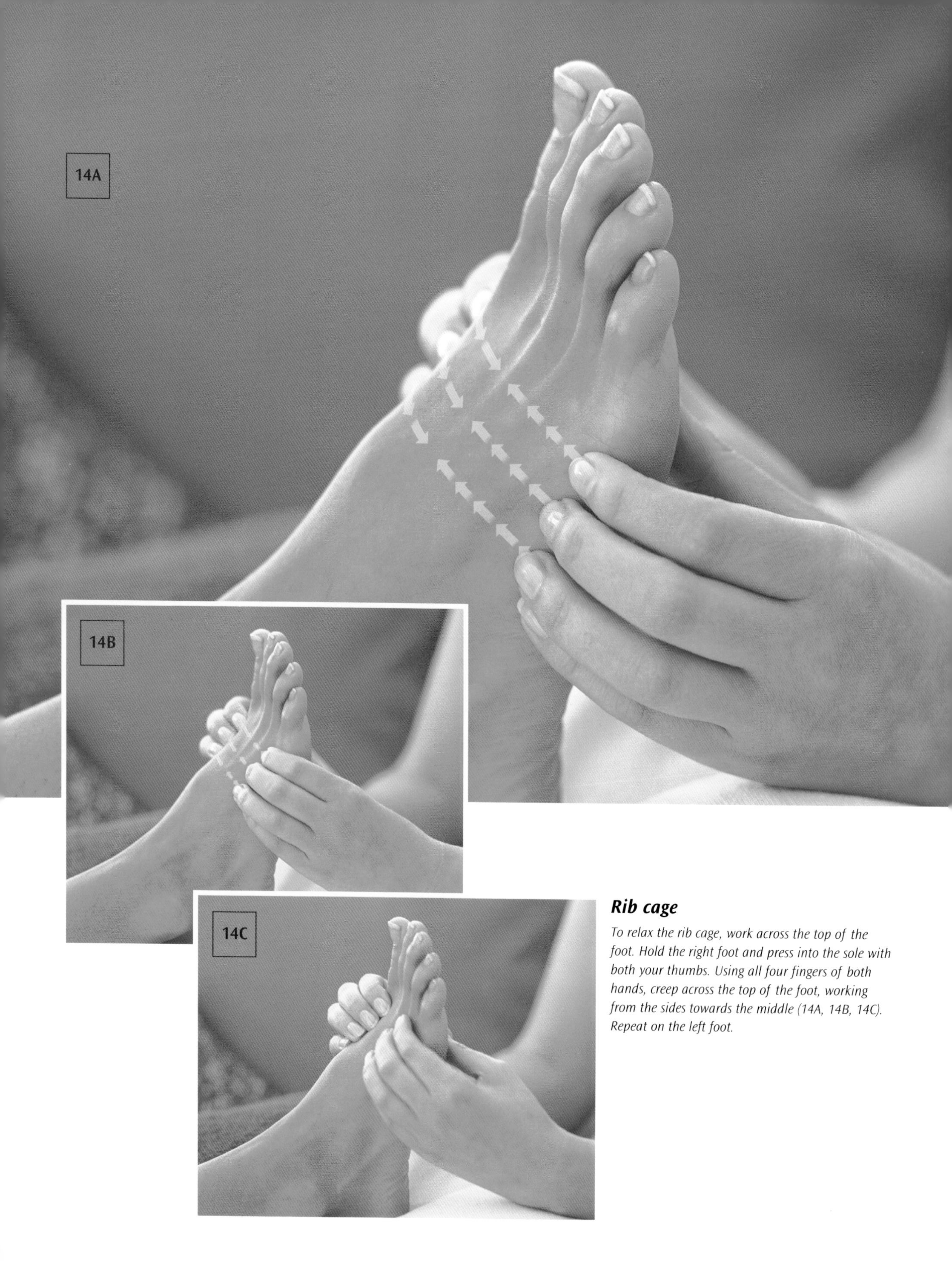

Rib cage

To relax the rib cage, work across the top of the foot. Hold the right foot and press into the sole with both your thumbs. Using all four fingers of both hands, creep across the top of the foot, working from the sides towards the middle (14A, 14B, 14C). Repeat on the left foot.

Self-help for back pain

There are reflex points in the hands as well as in the feet, but they are harder to isolate, since the surface area of the hands is much smaller. However, it's well worth trying this hand treatment for the spine, which you can do for yourself anywhere and at any time.

Rest your hand on a small cushion or pillow. Using the thumb of your other hand, creep along the whole spinal reflex from the base of the hand and up the outside edge of the thumb as shown (1, 2, 3). Change hands and repeat.

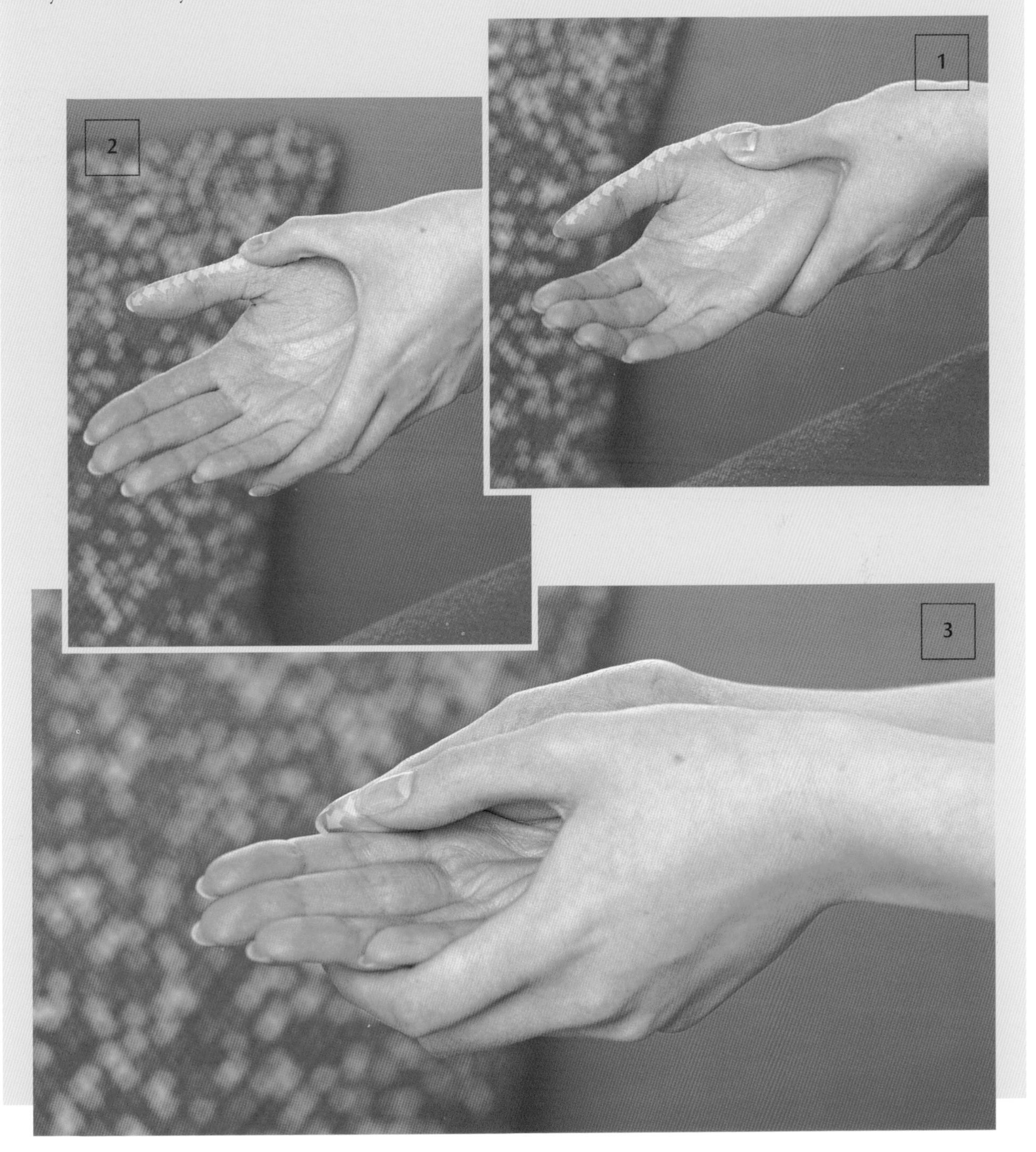

Useful addresses

If you'd like more information about reflexology or reflexology training, please contact the author:

Ann Gillanders
BSR (British School of Reflexology)
92 Sheering Road
Old Harlow
Essex CM17 0JW

Tel: 01279 429060
Fax: 01279 445234
E-mail: ann@footreflexology.com
Website: www.footreflexology.com

If you are interested in finding out more about aromatherapy, healthy eating, massage, homeopathy, naturopathy, or osteopathy, contact the organizations below:

AROMATHERAPY

The National Association for Holistic Aromatherapy
4509 Interlake Ave. N., #233
Seattle, WA 98103-6773

Tel: 1-888-ASK-NAHA
(or 1-888-547-2164)
E-mail: info@naha.org

HEALTHY EATING

National Nutritional Foods Association—Eastern Regional Office
136 S. Shirkshire Road
Conway, MA 01341

Tel: 1-413-625-8479
Website: http://www.nnfa.org/

MASSAGE

The American Massage Therapy Association
500 Davis Street, Suite 900
Evanston, IL 60201-4695

Tel: (847) 864-0123
Toll-free phone: (877) 905-2700
E-mail: info@amtamassage.org
Website: http://www.amtamassage.org/

HOMEOPATHY

North American Society of Homeopaths
1122 East Pike Street, #1122
Seattle, WA 98122

Tel: 1-206-720-7000
E-mail: nashinfo@aol.com
Website: http://www.homeopathy.org/

NATUROPATHY

The American Association of Naturopathic Physicians
601 Valley St., Suite 105
Seattle, WA 98109

Tel: 1-206-298-0125
Website: http://www.naturopathic.org

OSTEOPATHY

American Osteopathic Association/American Osteopathic Information Association
Chicago Office – Main Headquarters
142 East Ontario Street
Chicago, IL 60611

Toll-free phone: (800) 621-1773
General phone: (312) 202-8000
Fax (312) 202-8200
Website: http://www.osteopathic.org

Further reading

Craft, Drake, Dry, Ody & Van Straten, ***The Good Health Directory,*** Barron's, 2000

Von Cramm, Dagmar, ***Anti-Stress: Recipes for Acid-alkaline Balance,*** Gaia Books, 1999

Cummins, Shelley Lynne, ***Peaceful Journey, A Yogi's Travel Kit,*** Barron's 2001

Davies, Patricia, ***Aromatherapy: An A to Z,*** C.W. Daniel, 1998

Gillanders, Ann, ***The Busy Person's Guide to Reflexology,*** Barron's 2002

Gillanders, Ann, ***Compendium of Healing Points,*** BSR Sales Ltd, 2001

Gillanders, Ann, ***The Essential Guide to Foot and Hand Reflexology,*** BSR Sales Ltd, 1998

Gillanders, Ann, ***Gateways to Health and Harmony*** BSR Sales Ltd, 1997

Gillanders, Ann, ***Reflexology: A Step-by-Step Guide,*** Gaia Books, 1995

Lavery, Sheila, ***The Healing Power of Sleep,*** Gaia Books, 1997

Lidell, Lucy, ***The New Book of Massage,*** Ebury Press, 2000

Mabey, Richard, ***New Age Herbalist,*** Simon & Schuster, 2001

Mojay, Gabriel, ***Aromatherapy for Healing the Spirit,*** Gaia Books, 1999

Sands, Helen Raphael, ***The Healing Labyrinth,*** Barron's, 2001

Sullivan, Karen, ***Organic Living in 10 Simple Lessons,*** Barron's, 2001

Titmuss, Christopher, ***The Little Box of Inner Calm,*** Barron's, 1999

Wells, Judith, ***The Food Bible,*** Quadrille Publishing, 1998

Acknowledgments

Gaia Books would like to thank Lynn Bresler for proofreading and indexing; Bell McLaren, Kate Loustau, Sam Nelemans, Sarah Clive, and Suzi Langhorne for modeling for the photographs; and Jonathan Bispham DO (London) for his work on developing the foot maps.

Photo credits: All photography of reflexology techniques by Ruth Jenkinson

Other photography: page 12 Digital Vision, page 13 Photodisc, page 14 Paul Forrester

INDEX

Bold numerals refer to main text entries.

A

B

C

D

E

N

O

P

R

S

T

U V

W Z

A quick guide to the full routine

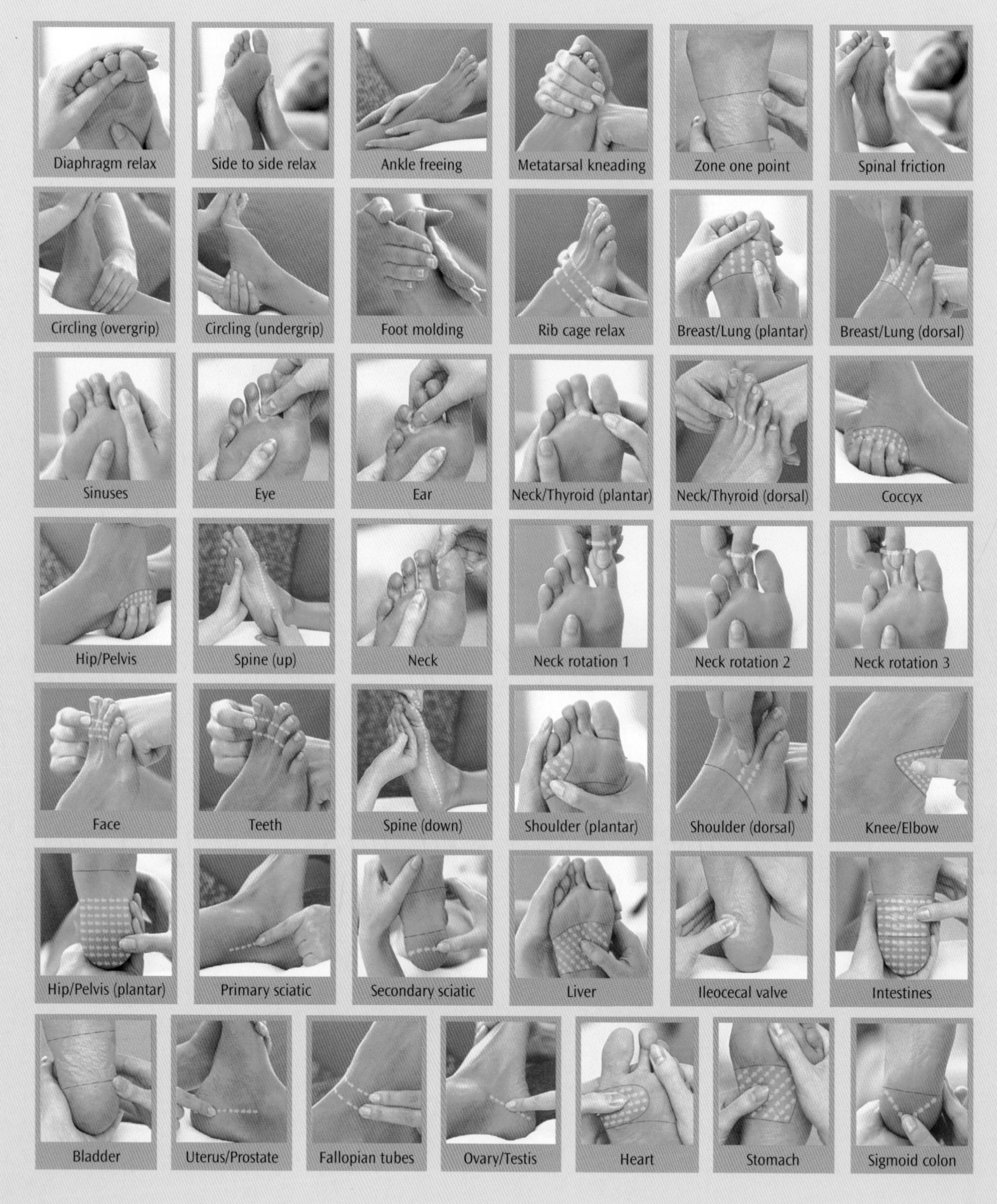